AF688635

NATURE TO THE RESCUE

Basic first aid using plants, food and spices

For novice and herbalist alike, Jessie has gifted us with a common-sense herbal guide to treating routine and 1st aid ailments at home! This book belongs in everyone's home as a useful reference for household health emergencies. Jessie has woven her medical expertise and herbal knowledge with grace and humor into a practical resource for all.

Susan Wayne Skelton

CFNP, RN, MSN, AHN-BC, Certified Clinical Herbalist, studied with Michael S. Moore

Jessie's work is without doubt an extraordinarily comprehensive and practical guide to equip ourselves with as we journey through our planet's uncertain future. The sections on first aid plants, radiation, and environmental toxins provides the perfect resources for my students who live off-grid and in very rural areas of New Mexico. The book is concise and well written, so that anyone from age 6 to adult can read and follow the guidelines and techniques shared. Jessie's work takes us back in time to the ancient knowledge of alchemy as she shares her invaluable wisdom and her expertise in herbs, along with the chemistry and power of plants, the first medicine in our world.

Kathryn Torralva-Villa

Science Educator and Curriculum Specialist for over 25+ years

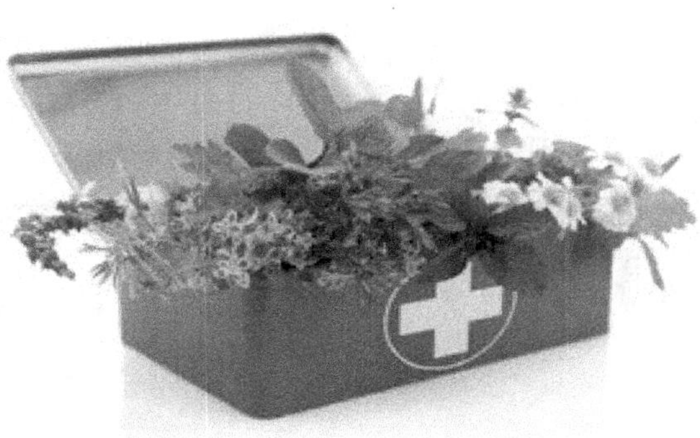

Using spices, foods and plants -
a Holistic approach to the treatment of medical emergencies and minor illnesses

"Leave your drugs in the chemist's pot if
you can heal the patient with food."
Hippocrates

BE PREPARED FOR ANY EMERGENCY
READ THIS BOOK NOW

Jessie L. Emerson RN, Certified Clinical Herbalist

AuthorHouse™ LLC
1663 Liberty Drive
Bloomington, IN 47403
www.authorhouse.com
Phone: 1-800-839-8640

Published by AuthorHouse 08/23/2014

Library of Congress Control Number: 2014907264

This book is printed on acid-free paper.

The purpose of this booklet is to provide basic information on first aid for some of the most common injuries and illnesses.

REMEMBER:

If symptoms persist or become more severe: SEEK PROFESSIONAL HELP IMMEDIATELY. The author and publisher disclaim any responsibility or liability for any loss that may occur as a result of the information, procedures, or techniques presented.

I DEDICATE THIS BOOK TO THE MEMORY OF MY DEAR FRIEND Phoebe Hummel whose artwork once again graces the pages of one of my books. We would go to the mountains and mesas together to gather medicine plants and refresh our souls.

It is also dedicated to the spirit of "freedom of choice."

A special thanks to Susan Wayne, RN, CNP, Herbalist, Jody Benson, whose expertise helped me in the process, and Grant Taylor, who stepped up when I thought all was lost. I just love Divine intervention.

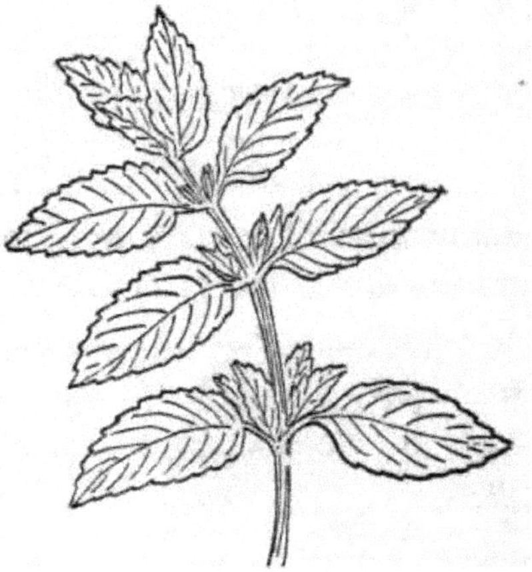

Mint, Mentha piperita

TABLE OF CONTENTS

INTRODUCTION
WHY AN HERBAL FIRST AID BOOK?

Herbal medicine is the oldest and most widely used form of medicine on our planet. The World Health Organization states that 80% of the world's 8-billion people rely on plant-based medicines for their health care. Herbs in general are simpler and cheaper than prescription drugs and have fewer side effects. This booklet is my personal collection of herbal remedies that brings together Western First Aid techniques and Western Herbal Medicine to create a holistic approach to treating medical emergencies and minor illnesses.

These remedies are based on the Western Herbal Medicine Tradition. In this regard, "tradition" does not mean superstition, but hundreds of years of developing soothing as well as life-saving remedies from the environment. I also offer remedies from my own decades of being a hospital nurse as well as a herbalist. My goal is to share the wisdom of these decades of using herbs and of learning what works and what doesn't. Some are folk remedies, some from my many herbalist friends, and some from southwest herbalist, teacher and author, Michael S. Moore. Although there are many herbal remedies, this booklet focuses on what can easily be found in an American kitchen, herb store, natural grocers, natural pharmacy, your back yard, and what you can grow in your own garden.

I believe that we must know what to do when there is no doctor and what to do until medical help is available. It is also important to know when to seek medical assistance. There are times when Western medicine and treatments are necessary. Reading this booklet can help you with emergencies, and help you decide when to seek a medical professional.

Jessie L. Emerson

Safety Rules When Using Home Treatments

WARNING: Never take essential oils internally. Even small quantities of some oils can be fatal

WARNING: Do not give honey to a child under 1 year old.

STAY CALM.

1. Knowing what to do before an emergency helps you stay calm.
2. Learn CPR and the Abdominal Thrust maneuver; take a First Aid Course.
3. Evaluate the whole person, situation, and circumstances.
4. Know when to seek professional help.
5. Know what to do until there is medical help.
6. Use information in this book as directed.
7. If you try a remedy and it doesn't work, try another remedy. Depending on the circumstances, you may need to *seek professional help IMMEDIATELY.*
8. Diabetics with foot injuries should see a healthcare professional immediately. Do not try to self-help in this circumstance.
9. Monitor progress. After a few days, reevaluate.
10. Stop treatment if there are any adverse reactions or if the treatment isn't helping.
11. Record keeping: Keep notes of remedies used and the outcomes, especially any adverse reactions. There is a space for notes in the appendix of the booklet. Keep a concise medical record on

self and family members. List the medications each person takes daily. Note any medication and food allergies and the reactions to them.

12. When in doubt, SEEK PROFESSIONAL HELP.

WARNINGS!

1. Honey is not for children under one year.
2. Pregnant women and children under the age of two years should not take herbs unless they are under the supervision of a person educated in using plant medicine.
3. Essential oils of any plant are never taken internally.
4. Do not exceed the recommended doses, duration, or uses of the plants. In other words, FOLLOW DIRECTIONS.
5. If symptoms persist or become worse, seek professional medical help.

Basic First Aid Rules

FIRST AID IS THE IMMEDIATE TREATMENT FOLLOWING ANY KIND OF INJURY OR MEDICAL EMERGENCY

WASH YOUR HANDS BEFORE AND AFTER WORKING WITH A PERSON. Wear gloves. Wash hands (for 30 seconds, getting between fingers and thumb and fingers) before applying gloves, and after removing gloves. Dispose of them in an appropriate manner. (See Home Medical Waste Disposal)

- **Stay calm,** take 3 deep breathes.
- **Assess** the scene. Are there any dangers to victim, bystanders, or rescuer? "Am I safe?" "What else could happen?"
- **Remove** victim from immediate danger: water, fire, smoke, carbon monoxide, gunfire.
- **Assess the victim.**

  a. Is the person breathing? Is it fast or slow, noisy, or quiet?

  b. Check for bleeding.

  c. Be aware of possible spinal cord injuries

  d. Is there a reason to suspect poisoning?

  e. Check for emergency medical information, e.g. Bracelet or necklace.
- **Initial Treatment**

  a. Maintain an open airway.

  b. Control bleeding.

  c. Keep warm and dry.

d. Give first aid for poisoning, ingested, inhaled or on skin.

- **Assess:** When immediate problems are under control, assess for problems that are not life threatening, heart, lungs, kidneys, diabetes.
- **Learn** exactly what happened. Could anything else happen?
- **How close is the nearest medical help?**
- Keep a list of emergency numbers on your cell phone.
- Know your capabilities, know when to seek medical help.
- **REMAIN CALM**

MEDICAL WASTE DISPOSAL

Use gloves when cleaning or disposing of materials that contain blood, chemical products such as herbicides and pesticides or possible infectious matter. Wash your hands before and after using the gloves. Use a heavy-duty plastic bag that has a biohazard label. You may copy and tape this biohazard symbol on the waste bag (zipped lock baggie). Color this Biohazard symbol RED to make it stand out.

If a person has a diagnosed infectious disease and is at home, consult the state health department for instructions that comply with your state's regulations.

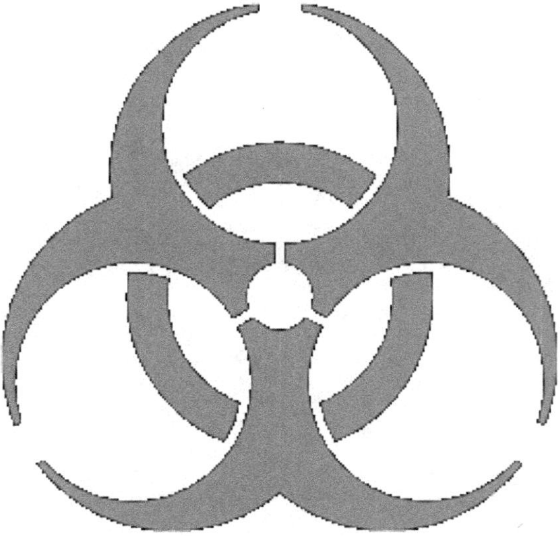

Prevention Is The Key For Emergency Situations

1. Poison-proof your home.
2. Know what plants are poisonous and unsafe for children and pets.
3. Learn the venomous creatures where you live, what they look like, their natural habitat, and the signs and symptoms of their bite.
4. Have an emergency plan for fire, flood, etc. and practice it.
5. Have a fire extinguisher in your home and car.
6. Keep Basic First Aid kits in your home, car, and backpack; a First Aid book is a must.

AILMENTS, EMERGENCIES, REMEDIES

ACUTE ANXIETY / PANIC ATTACKS; The out of control "fight or flight" response

Stop. Take 3 deep breathes,

Treatment:

1. Chamomile tea, a cup up to 4 times a day.
2. Passiflora tea, a cup up to 3 times a day.
3. Lavender tea, or apply lavender oil to temples, Smelling the oil is relaxing and calming.
4. Skullcap tea or tincture will stop mind chatter. Add 10 to 15 drops to tea or hot water.
5. Valarian tincture, as directed (the natural valium); this can make you sleepy so don't drink and drive.
6. Vinegar compress to forehead, useful for nighttime restlessness.
7. Bee pollen daily: DO NOT TAKE IF ALLERGIC TO BEE STINGS. Start with 1/4 tsp and gradually work up to 1 tsp, place in glass or cup and add juice. I add 1 tsp to my smoothie in the mornings.
8. B Vitamins aid and protect our nervous system. B Vitamins are lost during stress and high intake of carbohydrates. The vitamins in bee pollen: B1, B2, B6, pantothenic, biotin, rutin, folic, inositol, nicotinic, vitamin E, vitamin D, pro-vitamin A and vitamin C.

Acute Radiation Exposure

Unfortunately, this type of emergency does occur, has occurred, and continues to occur as radiation leaks at nuclear power plants, at laboratories, storage facilities, hospitals, and fallout from depleted uranium weapons. There is NO safe exposure or safe dose of radiation.

This book does not address acute nuclear fallout from bombs. Nor does it address chronic exposure from all the technology that surrounds us daily.

Prevention:

1. Do not build any more implements for nuclear war and disable those that exist.
2. Those who build and monitor those facilities must take responsibility.
3. Do not build any more power plants or weapons labs on earthquake faults.
4. Insist all uranium stays in the ground. That which is already dug must be neutralized.

Treatment:

Potassium iodine (PI) protects only the thyroid, but by flooding the body with iodine within a few hours after exposure, the potassium iodine can help crowd out the radioactive iodine to allow the thyroid to absorb the more abundant stable iodine. The children who received PI after Chernobyl have not been diagnosed with thyroid cancer. Those who did not receive PI have not been so fortunate.

1. Iodine dose as directed.

2. Have enough for all family members for at least two weeks.
3. The iodine in sea vegetables protects the body from radioactive iodine 125 and iodine 131.
4. Vitamin C, large dose up to 10,000 mg.
5. Miso broth several cups daily; anecdotally, it protected the patients who were at one hospital near Ground Zero at Hiroshima.
6. Root vegetables, and pumpkin
7. Sesame seeds, daily
8. Eat fermented foods: miso, tempeh, pickles, sauerkraut, red and green cabbage.
9. Soy foods
10. Cilantro
11. Strontium 90 tends to accumulate in cows' milk. Avoid cow's milk.

Acute Reaction To Environmental Toxins

Acute reactions can happen anywhere or any time. There are many chemicals in our environment. It could be said that we are a chemical generation. We come into contact with chemicals by breathing, touching, and ingesting. Our bodies react to even small particles of chemicals or radiation. Chronic exposure can lead to cancers and neurological breakdowns. Often, we may not know what the chemical may be. Acute responses are varied and depend on the chemical (s) and person. I have listed some common reactions.

Symptoms:

1. Chest becomes tight, difficulty getting your breath.
2. Audible chest wheezes or dry wheezy cough
3. Headache that becomes progressively worse
4. Irritated watery eyes
5. Runny nose
6. Nausea and vomiting
7. Rashes
8. Neurological symptoms: tremors, severe shaking, seizures
9. Asthma attacks may progress to respiratory collapse.

Treatment:

1. Remove from area causing reactions.
2. Open windows and doors
3. Drink cranberry juice, diluted with water for more palatability.
4. Powered vitamin C mineral drink
5. Cup of burdock tea neutralizes some poisons.
6. Cup of licorice tea soothes irritated mucous membranes.
7. Aloe vera soothes the skin, digestive tract and reduces inflammation.
8. Drinking green tea throughout the day reduces inflammation.
9. Lavender salve made with olive oil is soothing and healing.

10. Itching can be relieved with a cool compress of mint tea or mugwort tea, or apply a paste made with oatmeal and cool water.
11. Headaches usually clear when irritant is removed. A relaxing tea of chamomile will help, continue with the neutralizing remedies.
12. Cup of milk thistle tea will protect the liver and is recommended to drink daily for 1-2 weeks after the exposure.
13. These remedies are emergency measures. I recommend following up with a healthcare professional.
14. Document the episode: date, time, place. Weather conditions, name of toxin if known.
15. Be assessed yearly for any symptoms or internal damages and continue to monitor throughout the years.

Allergic Reactions To Skin Contact With Plants

Poison ivy, *Toxicodendron radicanes*, OAK, *Toxicodendron diversilobum*, or SUMAC, *Toxicodendron vernix*: These plants contain an oil that can be an irritant to some people. Even the smoke from burning plants is dangerous and can cause breathing difficulties.

Prevention:

1. Learn to recognize these plants and avoid them.
2. "Leaves of three, leave them be."
3. Wear long sleeves, long pants when walking where they are known to grow.

4. Remove these plants from your property or label them off limits. Do not burn them—the volatile oils can damage the lungs.
5. The oils of these plants can transfer to clothes, shoes, pets, and can stay potent for years.
6. Wash hands with soap and water; wash under fingernails.
7. Do not let water drip onto unexposed skin.
8. Wash clothes with soap and water.
9. Clean shoes; wash if possible.
10. Don't scratch; it will spread and cause an infection.

Symptoms:

1. Redness can affect eyes, mouth, genitals.
2. Itching may become intense and severe.
3. Swelling
4. Blisters may be surrounded by redness.
5. Difficulty breathing if smoke inhaled.

Treatment:

1. Wash within 30 minutes of exposure. Wash area with mild soap and water, taking care not to let water drip on unaffected parts of body.
2. Apple Cider vinegar: bathe area with it.
3. Aloe vera leaf: Squeeze the juice on area.
4. Paste of oatmeal made with cool water and applied will soothe.

5. Apply Paste of sodium bicarbonate, gently wash, and reapply throughout the day.
6. Green tea internally and as a compress helps inflammation.

Seek Medical Help When:

1. Itching cannot be controlled.
2. Rash affects face, eyes, genitals.
3. Rash becomes infected: pus, yellow fluid leaking from blisters, foul odor, increased tenderness or pain, increased swelling or swelling persists.

Altitude Sickness

Altitude sickness is associated with rapid ascent from sea level to 8,ooo feet. The symptoms are the result of decreased oxygen concentration caused by the lower atmospheric pressure at high altitudes.

The brain and lungs can be severely affected, and altitude sickness rapidly becomes **HACE**: High Altitude Cerebral Edema or **HAPE:** High Altitude Pulmonary Edema.

Prevention:

1. Start your ascent slowly, especially if going 18,000 feet or higher.
2. If you are taking heart medicine, blood pressure medication, diabetic medicine, have COPD, asthma, wear oxygen at night, have a pacemaker, come from a region that is sea level, drink alcohol daily, smoke anything daily, and your destination is 6,000 to 8,000 feet, have a conversation with your health care professional about your travel plans.

3. Build up your red blood cells before the visit/
    a. Dandelion tea, rosehip tea are iron and vitamin C in balance.
    b. Chlorophyll: 1 tsp. in 8 oz. water as directed. Do this daily for 1-2 months before your visit.
    c. Blue green algae taken as directed.
    d. If you smoke this is a perfect time to stop and clean your lungs. Mullein, Horehound, Yerba Santa, Osha, Horsetail, Grindelia strengthen and soothe the lungs.
    e. One book, Medicine for Mountaineering edited by James A. Wilkerson is a place to start learning about how to climatize yourself before going out and up.

Symptoms:

1. Fatigue, weakness
2. Unable to sleep at night.
3. Headache
4. Dizzy
5. Loss of appetite
6. Shortness of breath
7. Nausea and vomiting
8. These can progress to full acute respiratory failure, respiratory and cardiac arrest, and death.

Treatment:

1. Immediate and rapid descent to a lower altitude, at least 2,000 (610 meters)

2. Depending on the person and circumstances, a few days of rest may be all that is needed.
3. The extreme, evacuation to the nearest lower elevation hospital, oxygen, overnight monitoring

Asthma

Asthma is a potentially fatal condition. The lungs control the body's *CHI* or *Life Force*. Asthma is a condition in which the small bronchial airways constrict. The lungs don't get enough oxygen, which means the brain and heart don't get enough oxygen. Often eliminating white flour, white sugar, and dairy products made with cow's milk can eliminate attacks. The chemicals in cow's milk and the chlorine used to bleach the flour and sugar to make them white can trigger respiratory issues.

There are emotional and environmental components in triggering acute responses. The lungs and our emotions are closely connected. Learning to express feelings in all situations can help prevent anxiety and attacks of asthma. In our environment we are surrounded by chemicals and pollutants. Everyone is different and reacts differently to situations, chemicals, pollens, etc. No matter the cause, it is frightening to be struggling to breathe.

The rescue person must remain calm to help the victim remain calm. If you use an inhaler for emergency situations always carry it with you. Be aware of the expiration date—keep it current. Do not leave it in the vehicle in hot weather. If symptoms persist or are becoming worse, call 911.

Symptoms:

1. Breathlessness: breathing becomes more and more difficult.

2. Coughing: the body's attempt to expel irritants and mucus.
3. Audible wheezes: air struggles through the narrowed passageways.
4. Increased mucus secretions which further restrict the airways.

Treatment:

The goal is to relax the bronchioles, open the airways, soothe the respiratory tract, and calm the victim. If you or someone you know has asthma, ensure you have these herbs available.

Depending upon the person and situation, have them gently touch the back of their tongue with their teeth. This will help restore normal respirations.

1. Caffeine: Very strong coffee or expresso, strong black or green tea. This may not work if the person is a heavy caffeine user.
2. Chocolate: dark and minimally sweetened is good. Organic is best: 2 - 3 cups cacao or 1/2 ounces of dark chocolate bar, repeat as necessary.
3. Thyme tea is an expectorant and bronchial dilator: 1 - 3 cups as necessary.
4. Fennel: drink 1 cup every 1 - 2 hours.
5. Marjoram: drink 1 cup every 1 - 2 hours.
6. Ephedra: the American species of the southwest is not a potent stimulant as is the species from China, but it works very well as a bronchial dilator. Dose not to exceed 3-cups a day.

7. Licorice tea: NOT the gooey licorice candy one sees in stores. It the root of the licorice plant and is for short term use only. Long-term use can cause high blood pressure in some individuals. It soothes and calms the respiratory tract and supports the adrenals.
8. Mullein leaf tea 1 - 3 cups during the day. Mullein opens and soothes the tiny air sacs of the lungs. Remember to strain the tiny hairs using cheese cloth or unbleached coffee filters, and a strainer.
9. Horehound and grindelia are bitter and act as expectorants and help clear the lungs of mucus and foreign material.
10. Chamomile and skullcap relax the person. If the person can relax their body, they relax the lungs to make it easier to breathe.
11. Eucalyptus in steam inhalation helps prevent infection. Add 2 drops to 1-pint boiling water, remove from heat. Lean over the container with a towel to make a tent over you and the container. Inhale the steam.
12. Other plants for tea or inhalation: Mullein, Comfrey, Yerba Negrita.

If these treatments are not working and symptoms persist or become worse, medical help is imperative. The rescuer remaining calm is extremely important as a calming attitude can help calm the victim.

Athletes' Foot and Other Fungal Infections

Prevention:

Many fungal infections grow in a circle and often itch. There are other infections such as Fingernail/toenail fungus making the nails become rough and thick. With a fungal infection there is often head hair-loss. Fungi usually prefer warm, moist, or dark places. Often washing the infected part with soap and water two times a day is all that is needed. Keep the effected parts dry. Change socks and underwear often during the day. Expose the skin to sunlight twice a day for 5 - 10 minutes, although to avoid sunburn, avoid sunning between 10 AM and 3 PM on summer days.

Treatment:

1. Make a tea with garlic cloves:
    a. Mash 3 - 6 cloves.
    b. Pour 1 cup boiling water over them.
    c. Steep (let soak) for 15 - 20 minutes, the longer the stronger.
    d. Strain.
    e. Pour into foot bath.
    f. Soak 15 - 20 minutes
    g. Do this nightly. Dry feet, especially between the toes.
2. Licorice Root (not candy): add to garlic foot-soak, powder the root and sprinkle in socks.
3. Powdered marjoram: add to cornstarch and use it as powder in socks, change socks 2 - 3 times a day, wash, and dry feet, apply powder to clean socks.

4. Honey and garlic poultice to area 2 - 3 times a day.
5. Aloe Vera applied to feet after soak to sooth the feet, air dry.
6. At sock changes apply vinegar and let dry. Vinegar changes the PH, makes the environment acidic and unhospitable to the fungi.
7. This worked for me when I had a ringworm on the palm of my hand: After washing my hands, I applied fresh lemon juice (lowers PH) to palm area using a cotton ball 3 - 4 times a day. I mixed powdered turmeric into the juice to make a thick paste, applied it to the area, and covered the area with a large band aid. Within 2 - 3 days the infection was gone.
8. Other herbs that can be powered and applied or used in compresses or soaks:
    a. Tea Tree
    b. Chamomile
    c. Chaparral

Back Ache, Muscle Aches And Spasms

For movement to occur, some muscles contract, while others relax. Problems occur when there is over-contraction or over-relaxation.

Prevention:

Proper body mechanics for lifting:

1. Stand with feet pointing straight ahead, not turned sideways.
2. Use thigh muscles to lift, not smaller back muscles.
3. Squat and bring the object close to you before you lift.

Symptoms:

Pain: Muscle spasms, may be unable to stand up straight

Treatment:

1. Mix cayenne or red chili in sunflower or olive oil, apply to painful area. It will sting initially, but then you will be pain free for 6 - 8 hours.
2. Soak for 15 minutes in hot bath with Epsom salts and lavender. Do this one, two, or even more times a day.
3. Compress made from: clove buds, arnica, or apple-cider vinegar.
4. Teas for muscle relaxation: skullcap, chamomile, catnip, yarrow.
5. Use arnica liniment or salve.
6. Teas for pain and inflammation include: green tea, chamomile, vervain, aspen, and willow bark.
7. In acute stages apply ice or cold-water compresses for 15 minutes, then apply heat for 15 minutes, alternate until antispasmodics begin to take effect.

Bites: Human, Animal, Reptile, Insects, Spiders

DO NOT PANIC: The first rule in any bite is, DO NOT PANIC. The increased heart rate circulates venom quickly throughout the body.

Human, Animal

Human and animal mouths contain a variety of bacteria and viruses that can cause infections and death.

Prevention saves tears, time, and lives. Learn and teach your children how to be safe around animals, both domestic and wild. Know what poisonous insects and reptiles look like and where they live. Anyone known to have severe reactions to insect stings *must* carry epinephrine in a kit or an "Epi Pen". It is important to continue to monitor the expiration date of kit or pen. Always be aware. We share the Earth with other inhabitants. The sun shines on us all.

As with all wounds, be aware of the signs of infection. Inspect the area twice daily, in the morning and when you go to bed. Check more frequently if you think there is a chance for infection.

If after several days it doesn't improve or gets worse, check with your medical practitioner. Remember, wash your hands before and after applying gloves. Dispose of medical waste appropriately.

Prevention:

1. Teach children safe pet behavior. Never get in a cat or dog's face. Do not pull tail or ears, or poke or squeeze the animal's body too tightly. Teach children how to gently pet an animal.
2. When hiking: for safety with wild animals, do not let children or dogs run ahead of you. Keep your distance when you notice any animals; stay 300 feet away and do not chase or follow them. Do not come between a mom and her babies.
3. If you see an animal staggering, acting strangely, and/or foaming at the mouth, leave the area at once. With the possibility of rabies, it is important to call the local authorities so they can take charge of the situation.
4. Store garbage and trash away from house. Do not approach garbage and trash containers in sandals or bare feet. Plant tansy around compost and near trash containers to repel ants.

5. Plant plants that repel insects around play areas and the patio; even those that attract bees and other insects are better not planted close to people areas.
6. Carefully remove wasp nests from people's areas. Do not poke at wasps or hornets or harass them in any way. They have short tempers along with strong survival and territorial instincts and *will* attack. There are usually individuals or businesses who can humanely remove nests of these critical pollinators.
7. Do not put your hands into spaces where you can't see. Who knows what critter might be there? Spiders, scorpions, and snakes like dark sheltered places.
8. It is always a good idea to use herbal insect repellant when in insect territory. Do not wear perfume or strong scented lotions or make-up.
9. If you live close to wild animals, store pet food and birdseed indoors. Take in seed feeders and hummingbird feeders at night.
10. Inspect the body, scalp, and hair daily when camping or in known tick areas. Do this especially before you crawl into bed or into a sleeping bag. And make sure to shake out the sleeping bag first. The one time I didn't, I had an unplanned visitor. I was lucky it was only a moth.
11. Keep your tent zipped up when not occupied. Tents make nice cozy hangouts for critters. Before going into a dark closet, shine a light. Spiders like dark spaces. The black widow loves wood piles.
12. Some camping rules to avoid bear encounters:

a. Cook 100 yards from your tents.

b. When entering your tent for the night do *not* wear the clothes you cooked in.

c. Store all food in plastic bags away from camp: 100 yards and 14 feet up a tree, and 4-feet away from the trunk.

d. If you see an animal carcass leave the area immediately. A cougar or bear may be nearby guarding its food supply.

e. Never take food into your tent for a late-night snack. Bears like late night snacks also.

f. When fishing, do not clean the fish at or near your camp.

g. Bear pepper spray: Read the instructions and the expiration date. Know how to use it BEFORE you must use it. It is NOT a repellant, do not spray people, tents, camping equipment, or around the camp on grass or bushes. The spray is designed to be sprayed on the face of the bear. *Bear spray is not a substitute for common sense.*

Insects And Spiders

Symptoms:

Allergic reactions to a bite may occur within minutes or up to 24 hours. Mark on a calendar the day a tick was removed for possible future reference. Each critter and its venom have their own set of symptoms. No matter what bites you, ***start treatment immediately.***

1. Anaphylactic: hives, shortness of breath, difficulty breathing, swelling of tongue or lips, weakness, vomiting, collapse leading to death.
2. Fever, chills, headache, painful swollen lymph glands, malaise, collapse.
3. Painful blisters over body
4. Blisters forming around eyes, become red swollen, tearing, and light sensitivity.
5. Mound shaped red welt, the size of a quarter, very painful, ulcerated sore if untreated.
6. Cramping, nausea and vomiting, dizziness, difficulty breathing, weakness, headache.
7. Itchy red raised areas on skin; Be suspicious if you have pets. Fleas are vectors that carry a variety of diseases.
8. Plague: rapid-onset fever, chills, headache, muscle aches, malaise, nausea, painful swollen lymph glands, collapse.

Goals of Treatment:

1. Prevent infection.
2. If there is an open wound, pour water, flush with water for 5 - 10 minutes.
3. Wash the area of bite or sting with soap and water, apple cider vinegar, rehydrated antiseptic powder.
4. Bee sting:
    a. Remove the bee stinger: DO NOT squeeze, this will inject more venom.
    b. Lift off with fingernail or scrape off with knife.

c. Do not massage, rub, or scratch as this helps spread the poison.

d. Apply ice or wet cold towel to site. This keeps the venom localized while a poultice is being made. Remember to wrap the ice in a towel or layered cloth before applying.

e. Do not use heat, this increases circulation and spreads the poison.

5. Poultices are used to draw out venom or poisons. They may be applied until symptoms are relieved.

   a. Bentonite clay, baking soda, or soil (yes, soil. I had to use it for myself because nothing else was available; drew out the poisons, washed the dirt off with soap and water, and no further issues or infections—just relief).

   b. White bread, moisten and apply; change and reapply as needed.

   c. Prickly pear pad: remove stickers and peel, place slimy side down on area, change after 15 minutes, apply a fresh one as often as needed. I had this used on me when I received a bite or sting from an unknown assailant that produced a severe, immediate reaction. The pad was changed several times and was very effective, pain relieved and redness gone.

   d. Apply slices of raw potato, turnip, or cabbage leaves, change every 15 minutes,

   e. Plantains are found just about everywhere across the USA. It takes away the sting and pain while drawing out the toxins. Crush or chew to make a slimy mass, and place directly on site. Change and reapply as needed.

f. Pinon sap has both drawing and antiseptic properties. I carry the actual sap, and a salve made of the sap as a member of my personal hiking kit. If you are using the actual sap, place in a baggie or piece of cloth and soften it in your armpit so it can be applied. The salve works well!

10. Mosquitos, wasps, and chiggers: treat with lemon juice, apple cider vinegar, lavender, or cinnamon oil.

11. Black Cohosh helps the pain and muscle spasms.

12. Echinacea and black cohosh as tea or tincture are useful in any bite or sting, including a snake bite. Echinacea will detox and neutralize the venom and prevent infection. If you have a snake bite, stay calm. Start taking the echinacea internally, 15 to 30 drops in a 1/3 cup water every 30 minutes for two hours. Then take the drops every hour—hopefully while you are on your way to the nearest Emergency Room. It will not interfere with Western-prescribed medicine and should be continued.

13. Nausea: mint, ginger candy, or tea.

14. Pain or fever: Willow, aspen, or cottonwood as tea, with a little honey to taste.

15. Skin irritation, itching: honey soothes, heals, and prevents infection.

16. Comfrey, calendula, or lavender salve, aloe vera gel or fresh pad to soothe, reduce inflammation, prevent infection.

Infection:

As with all wounds be aware of the signs of infection.

1. Monitor wounds carefully, several times a day.
2. Be aware of how the person is feeling. Do they have pain? Is it increasing?
3. Do they have fever? Check more frequently.
    a. Dressings may need to be changed more frequently.
    b. Observations, monitor the wound.

Sign of Infection

1. Redness, swollen, hot to touch, painful
2. Red lines or streaks going away from wound.
3. Swollen and tender lymph nodes
4. Bad odor
5. Yellow, greenish, or greyish pus

If you think there is a chance of infection: If you see signs of infection, if after one or two days, it doesn't improve or gets worse, see a health care practitioner immediately. The key is prevention.

Signs of Gangrene: Seek medical help immediately.

1. *Very bad smell*
2. Brown or grey liquid oozing out, skin turns black, air bubbles or blisters.

Treatment:

3. Use warm wet compresses over wound to draw out infections.
4. Apple cider vinegar is an antibiotic that sooths, heals.

5. Teas and compresses: oregano, clove, lavender
6. Increase Vitamin C in your diet and take vitamin C up to 5,000 mg a day to help your immune system and prevent further infection.

Puncture Wounds:

1. Require immediate attention.
2. Wash thoroughly, apply a white-bread poultice to draw out the toxins that can kill. Seek medical help immediately.
3. Be prepared to keep changing and reapplying the poultice until you arrive at the ER.
4. When was your last tetanus vaccine?

For large wounds, abdominal wounds, gunshot wounds

SEEK MEDICAL ATTENTION IMMEDIATELY

Ticks

Removing Them Safely.

Summer months are prime tick season, especially when there has been a mild winter. In some parts of the USA where winters are milder, ticks reproduce at a higher rate and don't seem to die off as in harsher weather. Ticks can be anywhere, even in the desert. While camping at the Anzo-Borrego desert, I saw them firsthand. Wherever you are and one does bite you, save it in a glass jar. The doctor may want to identify it to see if it is carrying Lyme bacteria.

Procedure:

1. Wash your hands and wear gloves. Crushing the tick releases the Lyme bacteria and you could infect yourself.
2. Do not use matches, lighters, petroleum gel or kerosene on the tick. This may make the tick vomit the blood it has already taken, spreading the infected blood.
3. Gently swab the area with alcohol or apple cider vinegar.

Technique:

1. There is a special tool for removing ticks. I used one with my dog Sophie, and never left a head under the skin. Without the tool:
    a. Grasp the tick with tweezers where the head is buried in the skin. Pull out in one motion.
    b. After the tick is removed, swab the skin again.
    c. Apply an herbal antibiotic salve.
    d. Save the tick in a glass jar.
2. Note the date the tick was removed:
    a. Mark on calendar
    b. Observe site and the person for 32 days for symptoms of Lyme disease.

Lyme disease was discovered in 1982 and is named after the area of its origin, Lume. Connecticut. It is caused by the spirochete Borrelia burgdorferi. There is an early acute stage that occurs 3-30 days after the bite. This is where the disease is most treatable. If misdiagnosed it becomes persistent and chronic. Lyme disease is the great imitator. It can mimic many conditions including autoimmune diseases that can in turn affect all the body's systems. It is a complex disease that is treated with antibiotics and immune system support. If you think you may have been bitten by a Lyme disease carrying tick find a doctor who is a member of the International Lyme and Associated Disease Society (ILADS) and make an appointment ASAP. Early detection and treatment is vital to prevent future complications and death.

Symptoms:

1. Red bull's-eye shaped rash that increases in diameter
2. Chills, fever
3. Dizziness
4. Fever
5. Muscle and joint pain
6. Nausea
7. Severe headache
8. Stiff neck

Do not rely on home remedies if any of these symptoms occur.

Seek medical help, taking with you the body of the tick in a glass jar.

As with all wounds, be aware of the signs of infection. Inspect the area at least twice daily; in the morning and when you go to bed. Check more frequently if you think there is a chance for infection.

If after several days it doesn't improve or gets worse, check with your medical practitioner. Remember, wash your hands before and after applying gloves. Dispose of medical waste appropriately.

Bladder Infections

Cystitis: Cystitis is inflammation of the lining of the bladder. This is usually but not always accompanied by bacteria. Untreated it can lead to sepsis (infection of the whole body) and death, especially in the older adult.

Prevention:

1. Toilet hygiene: Women wipe from front to back. This avoids relocating e-coli to the bladder causing infection.
2. Go to the bathroom *when the urge hits*. A full bladder is like a bacteria hotel; they, their family, and friends like it there.
3. Wash hands after urine or stool elimination.
4. Drink eight 8-ounce glasses of fluid daily. This can be herbal tea (without sugar) or water with juice of lemon or lime. If the temperature goes up, increase your intake of water.
5. Be aware of how much sugar and meat you are eating. Excess creates an acidic environment, which creates inflammation that creates pain.

Symptoms:

1. Pain on urination
2. A sense of urgency
3. The feeling that the bladder never empties.
4. Urine smells strong.
5. Urine dark-tea color with mucus shreds.
6. Floating traces of red sediment
7. Fever, chills

Older adults may become confused, restless; this can accelerate to sepsis and becomes a serious medical condition that demands immediate medical intervention.

Treatment:

1. Water: eight to ten 8-oz glasses per day, helps flush bacteria.
2. Cranberry juice: pure, no sugar added, 6 oz, 3 - 4 times a day. (Can dilute with water.)
3. Parsley tea: 2 - 3 times a day, diuretic and balanced vitamins and minerals to assist the immune system.
4. Corn silk: A tea made of corn silk will soothe an inflamed bladder. Drink as often as needed. When I prepare corn, local and organic, I save and dry the silk thus always having some in case there is a need.
5. Juices: carrot, parsley, celery, cucumber, 2 - 3 cups a day.
6. Increase Vitamin C intake, 4000mg to 5000 mg. What you don't need you pee out. It also kills bacteria on contact—a winning combination!
    a. Sources of Vitamin C:
    b. Rosehips
    c. Oranges
    d. Apricots
    e. Red peppers, chili
    f. Orange-colored vegetables, carrots; a carrot-ginger soup works well.
    g. Broccoli, cauliflower

7. Echinacea as immune-system support and antibiotic.
    a. Use Tincture: 15 drops, 3-times a day.
    b. Tea, 1 cup, 1 - 3 times a day.
8. In the Southwest we have Osha, a tea from the root of the Osha plant. One cup 3 times a day serves as an antibiotic and stimulates the body's immune system.
9. If the infection is slow to clear up or becomes worse, it is the time to seek a medical practitioner.

Bleeding

This may be the most distressing to observe but usually simple to control. First, where is the bleeding? Is the bleeding from an artery or a vein? An artery rapidly spurts bright red blood. Blood from a vein is a darker red and comes out slower. REMEMBER, almost all-external bleeding, even an amputation or partial amputation, can be stopped with pressure.

Glove Your Hands If Possible

1. Hold direct pressure by hand over a dressing. This prevents loss of blood while allowing normal blood circulation.
2. Hold the pressure for 15 to 20 minutes, if you think you have held long enough, hold for 5 minutes longer.
3. Do not peek under dressing; this disturbs blood clots and prolongs the blood flow.
4. If blood soaks through the pad, do not remove the pad; simply add additional thick layers of cloth or dressings.

5. Unless there is evidence of a fracture, the hand, neck, arm, or leg can be elevated above the heart. This uses Earth's force of gravity to help reduce the loss of blood.
6. The pressure-point method (see below) is used if direct pressure does not stop the bleeding. Because this technique stops circulation to the limbs, it is held *no longer than necessary* to stop the bleeding. Continue the direct pressure and elevation. Reapply the use of the pressure point if bleeding recurs.
7. The pressure dressing is not so tight as to stop circulation. Observe frequently for blue fingertips and toes. If the victim is conscious, ask frequently if they have numbness or tingling in toes or fingers.
8. Observe frequently for signs of continuous bleeding: blood soaking through and dripping.

Pressure Points

Areas of the body where arteries pass close to the skin and over bones are called pressure points. Be familiar with them *before* you must use them. Pressure applied at these points can inhibit or stop the flow of blood. **These pressure points do not substitute for direct pressure and elevation.**

Pressure Points

1. **Brachial artery:** Runs from shoulder to elbow on the inside of the arm in the groove between the biceps and the triceps, about midway between the armpit and the elbow.
2. **Popliteal artery:** Behind the knee
3. **Femoral artery:** The groin area

Tourniquets:

Tourniquets are extremely dangerous and should be applied *only when there is a life-threatening hemorrhage, and only by a person experienced in the technique*. "Risk a limb to save a life" is the decision one must make. **REMEMBER, once it is applied you MUST seek care by a physician immediately.**

To Apply:

1. Wrap a strong 2-inch-wide piece of cloth around the upper part of the limb on the part just above the wound.
2. Tie in a half knot.
3. Place a short strong stick on it and tie a full knot.
4. Twist the stick just enough to stop the bleeding.
5. Write down the time applied. This is very important for medical rescue personnel to know.
6. Seek medical help immediately.

IF A BODY PART IS SEVERED

Do not attempt to replace protruding body parts back into the body.

Cover loosely with moist saline dressing.

1. Add 1 tsp salt to one cup water to make a saline solution like the body fluids.
2. Dip dressing or cloth into the water.
3. Wrap the body part in the moist cloth.
4. Do not attempt to remove a deeply embedded foreign object.

Herbs To Stop Bleeding

There are herbs that can stop bleeding. These herbs are ground very fine. Make your own formula, add two herbs together, add anti-inflammatory and wound-healing herbs. For example, Yarrow and Chamomile or yarrow and comfrey leaf. Place the powder in jar or tin. Label with name, what it is used for, and how you use it. Keep it where it can be easily found. Apply after pressure has been applied or apply and then apply pressure.

1. Yarrow
2. Alum root
3. Cayenne
4. Cranesbill
5. Desert lavender
6. Dried puff ball
7. Organic tobacco
8. Ephedra
9. Plantain
10. Shepherd's purse
11. Vinca
12. White oak bark

Treatment:

1. If another rescue person is present, have them call 911.
2. Proceed with stopping the bleeding.
3. Place in rescue position on their side, top knee bent, arm under head when under control.

4. Cover and keep warm.
5. Assess for any other wounds. If they can talk, ask if there are any medical conditions that need to be known.
6. Observe respirations at all times.

WATCH for signs of shock.

1. Rapid heartbeat
2. Shallow breathing
3. Pale face
4. Cool moist skin
5. Detached, semi-conscious awareness
6. Call 911 if you have not already done so.

Nosebleed

A nosebleed can occur for many reasons. Stay calm. Soothe and help a child to stop crying. Crying increases blood flow.

Reasons For a Nosebleed:

1. Medications, anticoagulants including 81-mg aspirin. Report to the physician.
2. Any injury to the nose, from excessive scratching to a punch
3. Allergies, excessive blowing
4. Certain cancers
5. Hemorrhagic telangiectasia, a hereditary blood vessel disease

6. Hot dry air: use a humidifier, add eucalyptus or peppermint oil for added protection and fragrance.

If a nosebleed occurs after a blow to the head, it may be a sign of a skull fracture. Stay calm. Seek medical help. Depending on the situation, place in rescue position on their side, top knee bent, arm under head, keep warm. Report to your physician immediately—don't wait for a 5:00 pm call. If your physician is not available, go to an ER.

Treatment:

1. Wear gloves.
2. Have the person lean slightly forward to spit out blood.
3. Grasp the soft part of the nose firmly but gently.
4. Hold for 10 minutes, then for another 2 - 5 minutes.
5. Do not blow nose, may dislodge the clot, and start bleeding again.
6. Apply witch hazel to a cotton ball, insert into the nose, leaving a tail with which to pull it out.
7. Keep in for at least one hour.
8. Use any of the herbs listed above that have been ground into a fine powder. Dip the end of cotton ball in water or witch hazel, then into the powder, insert into the nose, leaving a tail with which to extract the cotton later.
9. Ice pack across bridge of nose; frozen peas wrapped in cloth fits nicely.

Blisters

Blisters are caused by friction. They may come from wearing new shoes, ill-fitting hiking boots, or bunched socks. The rubbing can open the top layer of the skin; fluid enters the space under the layer, and a blister occurs.

Prevention:

1. Break in new shoes and boots a little at a time, especially before going hiking.
2. Properly fitting boots are a must.
3. Wear two pairs of socks when hiking.
4. Stop, rest, check your feet. If you see a red area, called a "hot spot" treat it.

Treatment:

1. Use a solid piece of moleskin.
    a. Cut a doughnut-shaped piece and place the hole over the center of the hot spot or the blister to surround and protect the blister. This prevents further irritation and will help keep the blister intact.
    b. Tape over the moleskin. Commercial foot kits may have adhesive on the moleskin that you peel off and stick on.
    c. Be careful not to contact the hot spot or blister.
2. Blisters are one of the ways the body protects itself. **Do not puncture. Do not open**.
3. The blister is like a band aid. It keeps bacteria out and fluid in. To prevent infection, leave the blister intact.

4. Check the blister and/or hotspot several times during the day and before you go to sleep.
5. If the blister oozes or opens, apply antibiotic salve, a doughnut moleskin around the blister, and apply a dressing to keep it clean and dry.
6. A person with diabetes needs to inform their doctor about the blister.

Boils And Carbuncles

Constant reinfection is a clue that you might need to assess your lifestyle and diet. Something is affecting your immune system. Sores that don't heal and frequent infections can be signs of diabetes.

Treatment:

1. Wash the area with vinegar and water.
2. Poultice
    a. White bread poultice: sprinkle a dash of cayenne or chili on bread, apply to boil 4 - 5 times a day, this usually opens and drains the boil.
    b. Flaxseed or fenugreek seed poultice:
        i. Boil the seeds. This will produce a gelatinous mass.
        ii. Place on gauze or clean cloth, squeeze out excess water.
        iii. Let cool.
        iv. Do NOT put directly on skin; the mass holds in heat.

v. Place cloth with the mass on the boil for about 10 - 15 minutes.

vi. Do this 4 - 5 times a day. This will open and drain the boil.

3. After the boil drains, wash with soap and water, apply antiseptic oils of either oregano, thyme, rosemary, lavender, or tea tree oil to area with cotton ball. Wear dressing until drainage completely stops. You can also use an antiseptic salve. Keep clean. Change dressing in the morning, before bed and as needed.
4. Don't forget to *wash your hands* and dispose of the infectious material appropriately.

Bronchitis

An acute or chronic inflammation of the mucous lining of the bronchial tubes. Thick mucus may plug the swollen irritated bronchioles making it difficult to breathe.

Treatment:

1. If you are smoking, reconsider how the smoke is irritating your respiratory track, causing infection, inflammation, or both.
2. Drink 8 glasses of liquids to help thin the mucus.
3. Fenugreek tea several times a day.
4. Licorice tea: **CAUTION: Do not use** if taking steroids or blood pressure medicine, drink twice a day.
5. Thyme tea or thyme honey: expectorant, disinfectant, soothing.

a. Soak 1-oz thyme in pint honey

b. Leave in a warm place for 2 weeks.

c. Strain.

d. Remember, honey is not for children under one year old.

6. Eucalyptus as an antiseptic in the humidifier to moisten and soothe.

7. Steam inhalation: peppermint, eucalyptus, chamomile.

8. Wild cherry bark: tea or syrup as an antiseptic that soothes and stops coughing. You can find wild cherry bark in commercial cough preparations.

9. Eating some garlic every day is a preventative. It is a treatment for lung conditions because it is exhaled from the lung and has sulfur components that kills organisms present in the lungs.

10. Osha root tea: drink 3 times a day, add a little honey to taste. Stimulates macrophages in the lungs, helps kills bacteria and viruses, assists the immune system, and is anti-inflammatory.

11. Chaparral tea: 1 - 3 cups a day. This may taste strange but if my young granddaughters could drink it, so can adults.

12. Horehound tea, 1 - 3 times a day loosens the thick secretions, making them easier to expel, and helps reduce the coughing. Adding honey makes it easier to drink and adds additional protection as honey is effective against staphylococcus aurous.

Bruises

If you bruise easily, consult a healthcare professional. You could be vitamin or mineral deficient, experiencing side effects from anticoagulants or baby aspirin, or have a medical condition.

There is no such thing as a "baby "aspirin. It stops coagulation systemically other wise a doctor would not order it. Determine the reason for bruising and then treat it. Do not stop taking your anticoagulated medicine. Talk with your doctor first and work out a plan with the doctor.

Treatment:

1. Eat or juice dark green leafy vegetables.
2. Eat or juice citrus and other fruits high in Vitamin C and folic acid.
3. Potato poultice: slice thin and place over bruise, 2 - 3 times a day
4. Cabbage leaf poultice: place over area, 2 - 3 times a day.
5. The traditional steak over the bruised and swollen eye: I really have never tried this, but people have told me it works—not for the cow, of course.
6. Arnica: Not for internal use. Use arnica homeopathic. Apply arnica salve or liniment directly to the skin several times a day.
7. If taking fish oil or Vitamin E supplements, stop for two weeks. Observe yourself, if new bruises appear, consult your PCP.

Burns

Most burns can be prevented.

Be Alert and Aware when around an open flame.

Keep matches and lighters out of reach of children. Teach your children how to safely use matches or lighters. Turn handles of pans on stove toward the back of the stove so children won't be tempted to reach for them. Don't use kerosene or other liquid flammables to light a fire; children watch and imitate, sometimes with serious results.

Treatment:

1. Immerse the burned part into cold water or flush with cold water immediately. Do not apply ice cubes directly to the skin.
2. Chemical burn: remove any chemical splashed clothing. Flush or flood the area with cool water for 30 minutes. Do not let rinse water get onto unaffected parts.
3. Leave blisters intact; they form a natural bandage to keep bacteria out, body fluids in.
4. Keep as clean as possible to prevent infection.
5. Never put grease, fat, lard, coffee, mud, or feces on a burn.
6. If you can remove them without impacting the burned area, remove any rings or shoes or constricted clothing; later there will be swelling that make it difficult to remove them.
7. If any clothing is stuck, do not try to pull off.

8. Give the severely burned person plenty of water. They can easily go into shock because of pain, fear, or loss of body fluids.
9. Know the signs of shock (see Shock).
10. If the person is conscious give them the electrolyte drink, “Rehydration” 1 cup every hour if needed.
11. Treat the pain.
10. Treat inflammation.
11. See a medical person.

Types of Burns

1. **First Degree**: minor burns, outer layer of skin is bright red and painful, i.e., sunburn. These can usually be treated at home.
    a. Cold water to affected area, or cold compresses, for ten minutes or until pain relieved.
    b. Cold compress apple cider vinegar every 2 - 4 hours as needed.
    c. Olive oil soothes.
    d. Aloe Vera: split open the leaf and apply the gel; if using commercial gel, make sure it is 100% aloe vera gel.
    e. Lavender oil, apply after using compress.
    f. Fresh cucumber juice, can't juice, apply thin slices.
    g. Fresh, live, unsweetened yoghurt will relieve the sting.
    h. Solution sodium bicarbonate (baking soda), dip 4 x 4 into solution and apply as often as necessary.

2. **Second Degree**: This type of burn makes a blister. Keep it intact. First-degree rules apply.

    a. Keep intact—everyone got that now? This is important!

    b. Olive oil, heat to boiling, cool, to room temperature, test on inner wrist, place on dressing and apply.

    c. Lavender, thyme oil, add to olive oil as a bacteriostatic.

    d. Add honey to antibiotic teas such as thyme, lavender, oregano, osha, and echinacea.

    e. Aloe vera gel: apply gauze dressing lightly, change daily. When my son was three-years old, he burned the palm of his hand on a gas burner in the garage. I split a leaf of aloe vera, applied it to his palm, wrapped in a dressing, and applied an ace wrap. I changed this once daily. It healed, left no scarring or contractures, and he was able to use his hand without any problems.

    f. Honey: cover area with honey to soothe and prevent infection, especially staphylococcus. Gently wash off and reapply twice daily.

    g. Tar burns: (Contributed by David, RN) slather on mayonnaise. The mayo disintegrates the tar and makes it easier to remove (this is often used in the ER).

3. **Third Degree**: Destroys all layers of skin, is relatively painless (at first), may look white or charred. Follow all the burn basics.

    a. Cover large areas with gauze that has been dipped in solution of sterile water, salt, and bicarbonate of soda.

    b. If the burn victim is conscious, give fluids and Rehydration Drink.

c. A limb can be protected inside a clean plastic bag.

d. Seek medical attention immediately.

Colds And Flu

Virus is the culprit, and there are 100,939,140 viruses on Earth (September 2013). Antibiotics are given only for secondary bacterial infections.

Prevention:

1. Stay home. Don't infect others, especially babies, small children, and the elderly.
2. Avoid large gatherings and crowds during the cold and flu season.
3. Keep hydrated.
4. Frequent handwashing is your first line of defense: after shopping, being in public, using the bathroom, coughing, before and after eating.
5. Garlic, onions, and cayenne included in the everyday diet is your herbal first line of defense.
6. Sneezing, coughing into your hands and then touching the eye can cause eye infections.
7. If you are getting more than two or three colds a year, your immune system may need help. The nervous system and the immune system are closely related. What is going on in your life? Are you upset or feeling depressed? I once had a client who every time she and her partner weren't getting along, she "caught "a cold. Things improved when they parted ways.

Treatment:

1. Ginger tea, add lemon and honey or drink the following tea every 3 - 4 hours:

    a. Grate fresh ginger root, 1 stick cinnamon, 1 tsp coriander seeds, 3 cloves, 1 slice lemon, add to:

    b. 1-pint water

    c. Bring to a boil, simmer for 15 minutes, strain, and sweeten with organic honey.

2. Make a strong ginger tea:

    a. Dice 1/4 of the fresh root, bring to a boil.

    b. Simmer for 15 minutes.

    c. Add to a hot bath.

    d. Soak for 15 - 20 minutes.

    e. Dry, wrap in a wool blanket or sleeping bag and "Sweat it out."

3. Onions: my mother, Dottie, always gave me little green onions to eat at the first signs of a cold. An old Missouri remedy is to steep a sliced raw onion in honey and eat throughout the day. You can also juice an onion and add the juice to the honey. Onions contain sulfur, an antibiotic.

4. Citrus juice to increase Vitamin C in your diet. You may need to take vitamin C tablets, capsules or powder depending on severity of symptoms. Take 3,000 to 5,000 mg. What you don't

    need you excrete.

5. Teas of anise, fennel, parsley, peppermint.

6. Carrot juice provides Vitamin A, the anti-infection vitamin.
7. Chicken soup, add 1 - 2 garlic bulbs, one onion, strain, and drink the broth throughout the day.
8. Vegetarian soup, add garlic which is the main ingredient.
9. Licorice tea helps boost the immune system.
10. Snack on handfuls of pumpkin seeds throughout the day, contain zinc to help the immune system.
11. Make tea from antibiotic plants echinacea or osha, and drink 2 - 3 times a day.
12. Willow tea: It is bitter but will lower fever and help the aches and pains. Add some honey to make it more palatable.

Constipation

Fecal matter moving slowly thru the colon, so slowly that water and often toxic waste is reabsorbed by the body. The fecal matter becomes hard, dry, and difficult to expel. The toxic waste can cause cell damage.

Prevention:

1. Daily walks or other movement activity.
2. Adequate water: eight, 8-ounce glasses of water or herbal tea daily.
3. Diet adequate in fiber to add bulk, retain moisture, and stimulate colon movement.
4. "Going" when you feel the urge.

Treatment:

1. Start your daily walks.
2. Water: 8, 8-ounce glasses of water a day, more if doing heavy activity and sweating, or if in a hot climate.
3. Fiber: whole grains (ditch the white bread habit), salads, raw foods.
4. Warm prune juice or warm water upon awakening. Warm fluids start the intestines moving after a night of rest.
5. Carrot, apple celery, or grape juice at room temperature daily.
6. Jethro Kloss in the classic Back to Eden gives this recipe: Bran water daily in the morning: soak 1-cup bran in 1-quart water overnight. Strain. Keep refrigerated.
7. Crushed seeds of fenugreek, flax, chia, or plantain (psyllium). Add 1 - 2 tsp to food. It is tasty in salads. When using this remedy drink plenty of water to keep the bulk moving. More than 2-tsp may cause gas, bloating, or cramps.
8. Chia seeds: a drink popular in Mexico is refreshing and adds bulk and liquid to the diet. It is made by adding 1-tsp chia seeds to 8-oz of juice such as apple, Guava, watermelon, or your favorite; let set, and enjoy the zip and energy it provides.
9. Puree 3 stalks of rhubarb (*the leaves contain high amounts oxalic acid and are poisonous*) add 1-cup apple juice, 1-tsp lemon juice, honey to taste, heat to boiling, stirring, remove from heat and let cool. Enjoy, both the taste and the results.

10. Last resort: cascara and senna are last-resort remedies and are not for daily use. Chronic use of senna an cause heart problems.

Coughs

Night coughs, night sweats, and blood-tinged sputum are serious symptoms and require medical diagnosis.

Prevention:

1. Cover your mouth when you cough to stop the spread of infection.
2. Teach your children these simple techniques.
    a. Turn your head away from people.
    b. Cough into your shoulder, the back of your hand or into a tissue or handkerchief.
    c. Coughing into your hand and then touching objects or people will spread infection.
    d. Wash your hands after coughing, sneezing, or blowing your nose.

Treatment:

1. Honey, lemon, and ginger tea. Drink as needed.
2. Anise tea: 1 - 2-tsp crushed seed added to boiling water, simmer 5 minutes, steep 15 minutes, add honey.
3. Thyme tea: Use 1 oz fresh leaves to 1 qt water. Soak fresh leaves overnight. Strain, add honey, and take throughout the day.

4. My mother, Dottie, used to rub my chest with Vicks VapoRub (eucalyptus salve), then cover my chest with a piece of flannel. She also rubbed the bottom of my feet with Vicks (she didn't know she was using reflexology).
5. Horehound tea: add sweetener. It is bitter, which is why it works so well in helping to cough up the sputum from the lungs.
6. Horehound cough drops: years ago, when pharmacies were called drug stores, among the remedies and candies would be a bag of horehound candy. As a child, this was my favorite remedy for coughs.
7. In the Southwest, we are fortunate to have osha root and the chaparral plant to use as teas or tinctures for colds and bronchitis. Some might object to their taste. However, when my young granddaughters got coughs and colds, they would drink chaparral tea and lessen their coughing time.
8. Slippery elm soothes the throat and helps eliminate the "tickle." Use as tea or lozenges.
9. Mullein leaves are made into tea or can be added to other teas. Be sure and strain the teas to remove the little hairs.

10 Cough drops can be made from these herbs: elderberry, ginger, licorice, anise, lemon.

11 Drinking adequate water helps thin out thick mucus that may be restricting the airways and depleting the body of oxygen.

Cuts, Srapes, Abrasions

Although it might appear to be minor, a minor cut can become a major tragedy overnight. The skin, our largest organ, keeps organisms out. When the skin is breached it is an easy pathway for bacterial invasion. Remember: *wash hands before treating the cut.* Apply gloves if available. Wash hands after removing the gloves. Discard gloves appropriately.

Treatment:

1. Flood the area or squirt gently with a bulb syringe or basting implement to wash out any foreign material. Clean with soap and warm water, rinse gently.
2. Wash with a solution of vinegar and boiled warm water: 1 cup vinegar to 1/2 cup water.
3. Apply honey and cinnamon, both are antiseptic, and honey soothes.
4. Apply any one of these salves or oils: clove, thyme, oregano, lavender, or rosemary.
5. Salves or oils of osha, echinacea, tea tree (melaleuca) are antibiotics.
6. Fresh garlic crushed is antibiotic (contains sulfur). It may irritate the skin of some people. If it does, wash it off immediately.
7. Fresh dandelion leaves crushed and mixed with water is soothing and an effective drawing-poultice.
8. Calendula and comfrey are soothing and promote wound healing.

Monitor any cut, scrape, or abrasion several times daily for any signs of infection.

Any person with paralysis, diabetes, or foot neuropathy needs to inspect their feet several times daily and at bedtime. If one treatment isn't working, change the treatment. It there's still no change, seek medical advice *before* infection. Becomes worse and spreads in the body. If you do have diabetes, do not try to self-treat. See your doctor.

Signs of infection

The key here is **Prevention**. Wash the area and keep it clean. Inspect the wound twice a day.

1. Red streaks going away from wound.
2. Swelling
3. Pain
4. Hot to touch (touch wearing gloves)
5. Drainage, yellow, green, gray

Diabetic Emergencies

Safety tip: Wear a medical alert device that says you have diabetes. There have been incidences when diabetic emergencies have been considered drunkenness and the person has died.

High Blood Sugar

High blood sugar occurs when insulin levels are too low to meet the body's glucose metabolism needs. It is often difficult to tell the difference between low and high blood sugar based on symptoms. The only sure way to know is to measure the blood sugar using a glucometer.

High Blood Sugar is Caused By

1. Rebound effect from insulin overdose.

2. Infection
3. Disease process
4. Extreme emotional or psychological stress
5. Onset can occur over several days, can progress to ketoacidosis and coma.

Symptoms:

1. Extreme thirst
2. Dry mouth
3. Flushed dry skin
4. Very frequent urination
5. Breath smells fruity
6. Shortness of breath
7. Loss of appetite
8. Nausea and vomiting
9. Abdominal pain
10. Rapid pulse

Treatment:

1. Insulin to lower blood glucose. Seek medical help immediately if there are no directions available or no available insulin.
2. Bicarbonate of soda, 1 - 2 tsp in 8 ounces of water to prevent or correct acidosis.

3. Replacement of water, sodium, and potassium. There are products of powdered Vitamin C and minerals or use Rehydration (in recipe section).

Low Blood Sugar

Low blood sugar occurs when insulin levels exceed the body's insulin needs. It is often difficult to tell the difference between high and low blood sugar based on symptoms. The only sure way to know, for sure is to measure the blood sugar using a glucometer.

Low Blood Sugar is Caused By:

1. Overdose of insulin
2. Delayed or decreased food intake
3. Increase in exercise following regular insulin or medication dose.

Symptoms:

1. Fatigue
2. Uncontrolled yawning
3. Muscle weakness
4. Tremors
5. Headache
6. Blurred vision
7. Difficulty concentrating
8. Nervousness, anxiety
9. Irritability
10. Cold sensations

11. Confusion
12. Hunger
13. Sweating
14. Cold, clammy skin
15. Pale skin
16. Numbness of the mouth
17. Tingling fingers
18. Palpitations, heart feels like it is pounding out of chest.
19. Very rapid heart rate
20. Shallow breathing
21. Loss of consciousness
22. Coma
23. Death

Very low blood sugar may cause you to not be aware of your actions or surroundings.

Let others know if you are feeling any of the symptoms, so they can help you.

Treatment:

1. Check the blood sugar for a base line.
2. Rapidly increase blood glucose levels by oral intake of fast acting sugars, juice (grape, apple, or orange) with added sugar, glucose capsule, hard candy, or package of sugar (I always carry two to three packets with me in my wallet for emergencies), wait 15 minutes and recheck.

3. Follow this with a protein snack.
4. Recheck in 20 - 30 minutes.
5. If the person is unconscious, they require injection of intravenous glucose. **IF A PERSON IS UNCONSCIOUS DO NOT ATTEMPT TO GIVE THEM ANYTHING BY MOUTH**. Seek medical help immediately.

Diarrhea And Dehydration (They Often Go Together)

I believe it is the body's attempt to eliminate poisons from the body. The main danger is dehydration, especially infants, young children, and the elderly. Without treatment death can occur.

Symptoms:

1. Loose watery stools
2. Gas and cramping

Causes of Diarrhea:

1. Poor nutrition: poor nutrition causes diarrhea, diarrhea causes malnutrition, we must stop this cycle. Proper nutrition is important in preventing diarrhea.
2. Shortage of clean, uncontaminated water. Unclean water contains organisms that cause diarrhea and disease.
3. Intestinal flu
4. Other infections in the body
5. Malaria
6. AIDS

7. Inability to digest milk and other dairy products.
8. Allergies to certain foods: babies are often allergic to cow's milk and some artificial formulas. Most commercial baby foods contain GMOs.
9. Side effects from some medications
10. Certain poisons: this may be from heavy metal contamination of the water or plutonium poisoning.
11. Laxative or purges gone astray.
12. Eating too much fruit, especially unripe fruit.
13. A baby is started on new food:
    a. Mash the food well and mix with a little breast milk.
    b. Start with very small amounts.
    a. The baby's body must learn how to digest new food. It's tough getting used to this planet. Go slowly.

Signs of Dehydration:

1. Thirst: In subclinical dehydration, thirst is often disguised by, "I am hungry." The next time you feel hungry, rehydrate yourself with water or herbal tea. Herbal teas provide a boost in vitamins, minerals, and energy.
2. Little or no urine; the urine is dark yellow. Without water our kidneys can't clean the waste products out of our body. Waste products accumulate, and we become poisoned.
3. Sudden weight loss: the body is made up of 75 - 80% water, our bones are 25% water.
4. Dry mouth: chapped lips are just one of our body's cries for water. Instead of Chapstick, drink water.

5. Sunken, tearless eyes: often people buy “artificial tears” for their eyes when maybe all they need is a glass of water.
6. Sagging in of the soft spot in an infant’s head: this is a dangerous sign, act quickly.
7. Loss of elasticity or stretchiness of the skin: gently take hold of the skin between two fingers. If when you let go, the skin does not immediately rebound to normal, the person is dehydrated.
8. Very severe weak, rapid pulse, fast deep breathing, low blood pressure, fever, seizures, weakness, mental confusion, loss of consciousness.

Treatment:

1. When a person is weak from dehydration, they may be too weak to care for themselves.
2. Offer sips of liquids every 5 minutes until they begin to urinate with light-colored, yellow urine.
3. Offer the person frequent feedings of the foods listed. They may be too weak to take much at one time.
4. Small, frequent portions along with frequent sips of liquids are helpful and will produce positive results.

It is also important to look at the cause of the diarrhea and treat the cause. Remember if diarrhea and/or dehydration becomes worse, seek medical attention. It may be necessary to give liquids and electrolytes directly into the vein, medication may be required. However, most cases of diarrhea can successfully be treated at home—If you know what to do. If the cause is contaminated water, medical help may be needed to kill the organism and its eggs.

When a person has watery diarrhea stool with or without vomiting, act quickly.

1. With children and the elderly, there is no time to waste.
2. Offer frequent sips of water.
3. Keep them clean and dry to prevent loss of water through evaporation.
4. A baby should nurse frequently. For the older child and adult, 8 - 10 glasses of water.

Give small portions of the following foods:

1. Mash ripe or cooked bananas, for the baby; add breast milk.
2. Applesauce (cooked) is a well-known folk remedy.
3. Well-cooked papayas
4. Blackberry and raspberry leaf tea: use 2-tsps to 1-cup hot water.
5. Black tea
6. Mashed, cooked carrots
7. Rice, oatmeal: if there is vomiting, rice or oatmeal water.
8. Cheese, if dairy is tolerated.
9. Yoghurt
10. Teas: ginger, mint, chamomile, will also help painful cramping. A little honey will give energy and is effective against staphylococcus organism.
11. Chicken or veggie broth
12. Rehydration Drink: It is wise to keep this mix in a jar and ready for instant use. If making fresh, add 3 TBSP honey.

Remember: Honey is NOT for children 1 years old and younger.

Dislocations And Fractures

A dislocation is usually more obvious than a fracture. It is the movement of a bone out of its normal position at a joint. When the bone is out of its normal place, it cannot function. An X-Ray is often needed to distinguish between a break, sprain, or dislocation.

Symptoms:

1. Compare with the non-injured area, does it look different?
2. Significant deformity, twisted or bent
3. Bruising and swelling
4. Unable to use the affected part
5. The injured area may be cold and numb, or hot and swollen.
6. Pain when touched or moved
7. Bone or bone fragments sticking through the skin.

Treatment:

Seek medical attention. Do not attempt to set dislocation or broken bone unless qualified to do so.

1. Remove tight clothing and jewelry.
2. Stop any bleeding.
3. Clean any open wounds, with soap and water, ACV and water, or alcohol, and apply dressing.
4. Immobilize the injured area; the splint must include the areas above and below the injury.

5. Do this only if it causes no pain or if you must move the person before emergency personnel is available.
6. If the injury is an arm or leg, splint in the position it is found, do not attempt to straighten.
7. Use the person's body as a splint: arm to chest, injured leg to uninjured leg.
8. Use folded towels or blankets.
9. Assess the condition of victim.
    a. Make circulation checks every 15 minutes for first hour until there is emergency help.
    b. Can you feel a pulse?
    c. Is the area warm or cold?
10. Always check for other injuries.
11. If you suspect the person has a head, neck, or spinal injury, leave them lying flat.
12. Minimize movement.
13. Keep the person comfortable; cover the body with what is available to keep them warm.
14. Apply cold compresses to minimize pain and swelling.
15. If a bone or bone fragment is sticking out, cover with dressing. Infection is a major concern.
16. Elevate the affected leg if possible.

Dizziness

Motion sickness: Dizziness is defined as unsteadiness. Vertigo is disorientation of movement when everything around you is whirling. Both cause falling and injuring the body. If it persists, consult your medical practitioner.

Treatment:

1. Ginger: drink ginger tea, carry candied ginger with you. Take the ginger 30 minutes before driving or being on the water.
2. Celery seed: chew or make tea.
3. Sometimes all that is needed is fresh air, loosening the clothing, a drink of water or juice.

Earache

When an infant or young child pulls at their ear, it usually means an earache. If you gently pull on the ear lobe, and there is increased pain, it is probably in the ear canal. If there is a sticky yellow-green discharge, there may be an acute infection of the middle ear. Earaches can often be prevented.

Prevention:

1. Teach the child to wipe their nose, not to blow.
2. If there is a stuffy nose, apply salt-water solution with a medicine dropper as needed.
3. Breast-feeding is best.
4. Do not let a baby fall asleep sucking on a bottle. The liquid goes into their ear.

5. Do not insert a cotton plug. Let the infection drain out.
6. Never put a stick, wire, or similar object into the ear. My childhood doctor, Dr. MacDougal used to say, "Never put anything smaller than your elbow into your ear."

Symptoms of Perforated Ear Drum:

1. Intense pain
2. Partial loss of hearing
3. Discharge of pus or blood, lasting only a few hours

Treatment:

Do not put herbal oil into ear or irrigate ear if eardrum is perforated or thought to be perforated.

1. Clean out the ear using a bulb syringe: gently insert the tip of bulb syringe and insert a few drops of water or peroxide. This will loosen any crusts and allow pus to drain. Turn the head gently to the side to allow solution to drain out using earth's gravity.
2. Irrigate the ear using bulb syringe:
    a. warm boiled water and cider vinegar, 1-tsp water, 1-tsp vinegar.
    b. Insert vinegar and water,5 - 6 drops, four times a day.
3. Apply garlic oil with a medicine dropper, 1 - 3 drops. Never put a clove directly into the ear.
4. Mullein flower oil, 1 - 2 drops, helps the pain.
5. Oregano oil, 1 - 2 drops, will help the pain and is antiseptic.
6. Teas: Chamomile, mint, drink to help calm.

7. Echinacea tea, 1 - 3 times a day or 15 - 30 drops of tincture, three times a day. This dosage is for adults only.

Eye Issues

Eye injuries should receive immediate attention. Even a small injury can cause blindness if neglected. Foreign objects may be blown or rubbed into the eyes. Foreign objects that appear to penetrate the eye should only be removed or manipulated by an ophthalmologist (eye doctor).

Foreign-Object Symptoms:

1. Burning sensation, scratching sensation, feels like something is in the eye.
2. Pain
3. Photophobia (extreme sensitivity to light)
4. Tearing, over production of tears

Precautions:

1. Keep the person from rubbing the eye.
2. Wash your hands before examining the eye. Use gloves if available.
3. Copious irrigation: use 1 tsp salt to 1 cup boiled and cooled water.
4. Removing object from surface of eye or inner surface of eyelid:
    a. Pull down the lower lid to see if the object is on the inner surface of the lid.

b. If the object is on the inner surface, lift it gently with the corner of a clean handkerchief or paper tissue. Never use dry cotton around the eye. Moisten a cotton tip (use sterile water).

c. Have the person close their eyes and look to the left, the right and up and down. This will produce more tears and often a speck of dirt will wash out with the tears.

d. Gently pull the upper lid forward and down over the lower lid; tears may dislodge the object.

e. If the object remains, look to see if the particle is under the upper lid. Look for it by turning the lid up over a thin stick--like a matchstick. Have the person look down while you do this.

If after the object is removed, the eye still feels scratchy, there may be a corneal abrasion. Using an eye patch, cover the eye for 24 hours. ***NEVER*** *cover an eye that has a discharge or pus.* When the patch is removed, if the eye does not appear normal, seek medical attention.

If the object cannot be removed, apply a dry protective dressing, and consult a physician.

Blunt Trauma to Eye

1. Wash hands and put on gloves before examining the eye.
2. Treat with ice pack.
3. Keep person lying flat.
4. Cover with a dry sterile dressing or eye patch.
5. Seek medical help immediately.

Chemical Burns: NO Time to Waste!

1. Immediate irrigation is essential!
2. Irrigate for 30 minutes using clean sterile water if available.
3. Identify the chemical, alkali is more serious than acid.
4. Seek medical attention immediately.

Pink Eye, Conjunctivitis:

This infection of the eye surface is highly contagious. To prevent the spread among children:

1. Do not let a child with pink eye play or sleep with other children.
2. Do not let the child use the same towel as other family members.
3. It is usually self-limiting in two weeks.

Causes:

Bacteria:

1. Generalized reddened look
2. Scratchy eyes
3. Discharge is pus
4. Matted shut after sleeping
5. Discomfort
6. Sensitive to light

Virus:

1. Whites of eyes have blotchy red appearance.

2. Discharge is watery, stringy.
3. Discomfort
4. Sensitive to light

Allergic:

1. Faint red or pinkish color
2. Discharge is clear.
3. Itchy eyes
4. May have runny nose and sinus infection

Treatment:

1. Wash hands before and after working with the eye. Use gloves if available. By now you know it is proactive and necessary to have gloves with you in the home, in the car, and in your backpack.
2. Check eye to make sure foreign body isn't causing the symptoms.
3. Irrigate the eye with fresh isotonic water four to six times a day using a fresh batch of isotonic water each time.

Isotonic solution:

Isotonic solution is salt neutral. It matches our body. It is neither too salty nor not salty enough. With too much salt the cells dehydrate and shrink; too little and they swell and burst.

To make isotonic solution:

1. Use sterile distilled water or boiled water.
2. 1 rounded teaspoon of salt for 1-quart water.

3. 1/2 teaspoon per pint.
4. 1/4 teaspoon per 8-ounce cup.
5. Dip a cotton ball into the solution and drip the fluid into the eye.
6. Irrigate from inner eye to outer aspect to avoid contaminating with fresh bacteria.
7. Use a different cotton ball each time.
8. **Do this 1 - 3 times at each irrigation.**

Soothing pain:

1. A warm compress of aloe vera juice is soothing and antibiotic.
2. Add antibiotic spices to food: bay leaf, cinnamon, cloves, garlic, lavender, turmeric.
3. Anti-inflammatory teas: green tea, licorice.
4. If eye doesn't improve or gets worse:
    a. increased pain,
    b. increased swelling and redness,
    c. increased pus or watery discharge,
    d. decreased vision,
5. **See a health care practitioner immediately. Sight is more precious than gold.**

Fainting

Fainting is a partial or complete loss of consciousness due to a reduced supply of blood to the brain for a short time. There are many causes: hunger, low blood sugar, exhaustion, severe emotional upset, pain, and centuries ago, a tight corset. To prevent loss of consciousness and fall injuries, any person who feels weak and dizzy should sit down and bend their head down to the level of the knees.

Signs and Symptoms:

1. Extreme paleness
2. Sweating
3. Coldness of the skin
4. Dizziness
5. Numbness and tingling of the hands and feet
6. Nausea
7. Vision disturbances

Treatment:

1. Ease the victim to the ground.
2. If they have fallen, leave them there.
3. Turn them onto their side, turn head to the side.
4. Loosen constrictive clothing.
5. Bathe the face with a cool cloth.
6. Oil of peppermint, eucalyptus, rosemary, or lavender under the nose.
7. Teas when conscious: peppermint, ginger, lavender
8. Do not give any liquids if the person is unconscious.

9. Examine the victim carefully to see if they have suffered an injury from falling.
10. Unless recovery is prompt, seek medical assistance.
11. Because fainting may be part of the development of a serious disease, the person should consult a medical professional.

Falls

In a fall a person's full weight will go to the points of contact. This can cause tissue, organ or bone injury with swelling and pain. If the fallen person cannot immediately get up, the consequences can go from minor to severe. Prevention is the key.

Prevention:

1. Be alert and aware of your surroundings.
2. In your home keep pathways uncluttered and well lit.
3. Remove or secure throw rugs.
4. Pick up toys, both those belonging to kids and pets.
5. Use night lights, motion lights are helpful.
6. Be aware of where you place your feet, especially when hiking or on unfamiliar territory.
7. Maintain your strength and balance. Do daily exercises for strength, balance, and strong bones.
8. Maintain adequate hydration. Not drinking adequate fluids can cause mental changes, confusion, physical weakness, and low blood pressure. **DRINK UP SO YOU CAN STAY UP**.

9. Intoxication from whatever form, such as prescription medications (both legal and illegal), alcohol, and herbal intoxicants, they make you less aware and effect your balance.

Exercises to Prevent Falls

I found these exercised on the web site of the American Academy of Orthopedic Surgeons. These are to strengthen and maintain flexibility. If you are recovering from an injury, consult with your health care professional before doing these exercises.

1. STRETCH, your calf and Achilles tendon. "Stand close to a solid support and lean on it with your forearms. rest your head on your hands. Bend one leg and place your foot on the ground in front of you, with the other leg straight behind. slowly move your hips forward, keeping your lower back flat. Do your stretches slowly and gently. Do not bounce. Inhale as you move forward into your stretches. Hold breath 10 to 30 seconds. Then exhale and relax. If this causes pain, take your stretches easier, start by holding for 10 seconds and working your way up to 30 seconds. Be gentle with yourself.

b. BALANCE, "Stand on one foot with your eyes closed. Do this as long as you can, gradually build up to 30 seconds. Do this 3-4 times a day." Remove or secure throw rugs.

c. STRENGTHEN, "From a standing position, push through the toes of both feet and raise the heels off the floor while I could feel a difference in my balance and flexibility after doing these several times a day after even just one week. It does take determination and a willingness to do these each day. On the other hand, I don't want to fall, sprain an ankle, or break a bone.

Treatment:

1. Before you get up do a total body inventory.
2. If you are injured or feel severe pain, don't try to get up by yourself (unless in immediate environmental danger). You may create further trauma to yourself.
3. Call for help. Make yourself heard in any way possible.
4. Getting up slowly and correctly can prevent further injury.
5. If there are injuries, refer to other conditions in this book.

How to Get Up from a Fall

1. Roll over onto your side by turning your head in the direction you are trying to roll.
2. Roll your shoulders, arm, hips and finally your leg.
3. Push your upper body up.
4. Lift your head and pause for a few minutes to steady yourself.
5. Slowly get up on your hands and knees and crawl to something sturdy. If at home use a chair.
6. Put your hands on the seat of the chair; slide one foot forward so your foot is flat on the floor.
7. Keep the other leg bent with the knee on the floor.
8. In this kneeling position slowly rise and turn your body to sit in the chair.
9. Sit for a few minutes before you try to do anything.

Fever

Fever is a sign of illness. High fever is dangerous, especially in infants, small children, and the elderly.

Do not give children aspirin; salicylates in their isolated, concentrated form can cause a syndrome called Reyes Syndrome. Reyes syndrome can cause irreversible brain damage. If the fever is over 103, persists for over two days, seek medical assistance.

Treatment:

1. Do not bundle up a person with a fever. The less clothing the better. A tepid water bath, sponge bath, or wet, cool towels applied to the neck and chest will lower the temperature. If camping or hiking, wet your neck bandana and rewrap it around your neck.
2. Drink plenty of fluids, primarily water, and herbal teas. If the urine becomes scant or concentrated, increase liquids.
3. Ginger tea: drink to induce sweating. Pour a strong infusion into a bath of tepid water. Use as cold compress. Apply until fever breaks.
4. Peppermint tea.
5. Add cinnamon to teas for its antibacterial properties.
6. Elder flower tea: the German Commission E endorses using 2 to 3 cups a day for feverish chills. For taste, calming, and anti-infection qualities add chamomile to the brew. Peppermint can also be added.
7. Willow bark is a time-tested remedy, (Aspirin was created from the chemical compound in willow and meadowsweet by the Bayer company in 1830). It is bitter; use with

cinnamon, ginger, or chamomile and adding a little honey helps the medicine to go down.

Frostbite

This is the result of frozen cells and tissues. The nose, cheeks, ears, fingers, and toes are most affected.

Prevention:

1. Use the "buddy "system. You and your buddy check each other's face often during outdoor snow activities.
2. If alone, cover your nose and exposed facial areas.

Signs and Symptoms:

1. The area may become slightly flushed, later changing to white or grayish yellow.
2. Loss of feeling in hands or feet.
3. May have pain in the beginning but often it subsides.
4. The victim may be unaware of his frostbite until he sees the pale, glossy skin.
5. Weakness, staggering gait, falls.
6. Failing eyesight.
7. Unconsciousness.
8. Shock.
9. Stop Breathing.
10. Death due to heart failure.

Treatment:

The object is to prevent further damage and to warm the affected area rapidly, maintain respirations and prevent refreezing.

1. DO NOT rub the injury with snow.
2. Do not rub the affected part at all, may cause gangrene (death of tissue).
3. Do not drink alcoholic beverages.
4. Do not smoke. Do not smoke anything!
5. Do not attempt to thaw a deep frostbite if you are not close to medical care. If thawed and refrozen will cause more damage leading to amputations.
6. Do not apply heat lamps or hot water bottles.
7. DO cover the frozen part, provide extra blankets.
8. Do give the victim a warm drink, a little cayenne in hot cocoa will get the circulation going, as will peppermint tea and ginger tea.
9. Do immerse the effected part in warm water:
    a. Between 99' to 102°F.
    b. Take out of water immediately when becomes flushed (this indicates blood is returning to the tissues).
    c. Gently pat dry.
    d. Place sterile gauze between the fingers and toes.
    e. Keep these areas dry as much as possible.
    f. The areas will swell and may blister.

10. After the feet are thawed, do not let the victim walk on them.
11. Do have them wiggle fingers and toes to increase circulation.
12. Do Prevent re-freezing.
13. Do continually access the victim and treat accordingly.
14. Take the victim to the nearest medical facility ASAP.

Hangover

I debated with myself whether to include this malady. However, it happens often enough to warrant inclusion. Too much alcohol causes dehydration, low blood sugar, irritation of the lining of the digestive track, mineral depletion, acid build-up in the blood, blood-vessel dilation triggering headache and nerve pain. Prevention is wisest and best.

Treatment:

1. Water, water, and water, at least 10 glasses; if hangover is severe, add honey and lemon juice.
2. Juice: carrot, tomato, celery, onion, cayenne, garlic, black pepper. If only canned vegetable juice is available, add garlic, cayenne, black pepper. Drink throughout the day to provide minerals and vitamins lost from alcohol metabolism.
3. Peppermint tea.
4. Black tea.
5. Onion soup made with miso and add, guess what—garlic, black pepper, and cayenne. Drink 1 - 2 cups or until symptoms are relieved.

Headache

Everyone gets a headache now and again. About 90% are caused by tension. The other 10% are migraines, cluster, and caffeine withdrawal. If you suffer from migraines, note the foods you ate the day before and what chemicals you may have ingested or inhaled. Read the labels. There may be chemical additives in foods that trigger migraines. If headaches become chronic or severe, seek professional advice. For the occasional simple headaches try relaxation techniques, deep breathing, and visualization.

Treatment:

1. Water: our best medicine, drink your 8 glasses daily to prevent headaches.
2. Garlic, onions, and cayenne daily in your diet.
3. Chamomile tea to release tension.
4. Lemon balm tea for relaxation.
5. Ginger tea at onset of migraine, and then as needed.
6. Peppermint oil, lavender oil, thyme oil, rosemary oil applied to temples.
7. Relaxing hot bath at the onset, ginger tea or lavender tea or oil or Epsom salts can be added.
8. Thyme tea, hot compress applied to neck and shoulder muscles.
9. Cinnamon, peppermint, and rosemary tea.
10. Bay leaf, basil, sage tea.
11. A New Mexico treatment is a bandana soaked in apple cider vinegar and wrapped around the forehead. You can

also add thin slices of white potatoes soaked in vinegar to add to the bandana wrap.

12. This combination of juices has been found to help some migraines: carrot, spinach, celery, parsley.
13. Caffeine: strong coffee or black tea taken at onset. This is only effective if the person is not a heavy coffee drinker.
14. Feverfew has been used for centuries to prevent migraines and to relieve them. It is a smooth muscle relaxer and is antiseptic and can be used to wash wounds. It is available as tea, tincture, capsules.

CAUTION: Pregnant women should not take feverfew as it could trigger miscarriage. Nursing mothers should not take it as it may cross over to the baby through the milk.

There is some research that suggests magnesium deficiency may cause headaches. Look at your diet. Too much sugar and too little green "leafies?" Reconsider what you are eating. Purslane, green beans, peas, spinach, lambs' quarters, and other wild greens contain magnesium.

Heart Attack

This is a life-threatening situation. Call 911 immediately. It is my belief that everyone should know CPR. It could save a life, including one you love.

Cautions:

1. It is imperative to know the symptoms of a heart attack.
2. Not all people experience severe chest pain.

3. 65% of those who have had a heart attack had mild symptoms or symptoms that come and go.
4. Call 911 if you think you might be having a heart attack.
5. Getting help immediately or within 1 - 2 hours of when the symptoms started can save a life.
6. If the person resists and says they will feel better if they lie down, call 911 anyway.
7. Do not let a person drive themselves to the emergency room. They may go unconscious and fatally injure another.

Symptoms:

1. Persistent chest pain, usually under the sternum (breastbone)
2. The pain often radiates to one or both shoulders or arms, or elbow, or the neck or jaw or both.
3. The pain may be very severe or mild. The degree of pain is not an indication of the seriousness of the disease.
4. Gasping, shortness of breath.
5. Indigestion, nausea and vomiting, flu like symptoms.
6. Extreme pallor or bluish discoloration of the lips, skin, and fingernail beds.
7. Weak rapid pulse
8. Cold sweat
9. Pale cold, clammy skin
10. Blood pressure low
11. Weakness
12. Mental confusion

What to do:

1. Place a person in a comfortable position, usually sitting up. If extreme shortness of breath, use as many pillows as needed.
2. Loosen constrictive clothing.
3. Call 911 for an ambulance.
4. If the person has prescribed medication for chest pain, give as directed and note time and response.

Do Not Delay!

1. The person needs the technology and care of EMS and the Emergency Room.
2. Never give liquids to an unconscious victim.
3. Start CPR if the person is not breathing and has no pulse.

These measures are for comfort control only.

1. **Cayenne tea**
    a. If the person is conscious, give them a cup of cayenne tea to dilate the coronary arteries to send more blood and oxygen to the heart. This can decrease pain.
    b. 1/2 tsp cayenne in 1 cup
    c. Add boiling water.
    d. Let set until cool enough to sip.
    e. Do not attempt to drink the whole cup at one time.
2. **Tincture of Hawthorn and Cayenne,**
    a. Place 5 - 10 drops in 1/3 glass of water.

b. Repeat as needed.

Heat Exhaustion, Heat Stroke, Sun Tips

Heat exhaustion and heat stroke are two serious and potentially fatal conditions that can be prevented. Young children, toddlers, babies, and the elderly are the most affected. Follow these sun tips and enjoy the day.

Sun tips

1. Although we are dependent on our sun for Vitamin D and life, we must also be aware of the dangers of the sun's rays' UVA, the aging ray.
   a. UVA are intense dawn to dusk even with clouds.
   b. UVA penetrates to the lower layers of skin and interferes with collagen and elastin production.
2. UVB, The burning ray. Strongest at midday
3. UVC, filtered by ozone layer (if there is one)
4. All the rays are stronger in the mountains than at lower altitudes.
5. They are all associated with:
   a. Premature aging
   b. Weakened immune system.
   c. Skin cancers

Prevention:

1. Wear a hat with brim, especially if thinning or no hair. Heat is both lost and absorbed through the crown of the head.

2. Minimize sun exposure between 10:00 AM and 3:00 PM when UVB rays are the strongest. Children should play in the shade during these times. For adults it is equally inadvisable to run, jog, or mow the grass in peak sun.
3. The higher the elevation, the faster you burn. Water, cement, and snow reflect the sun.
4. Wear a long-sleeved shirt and sunglasses when in those environments.
5. You need more water with heat and sun exposure. Drink water before exercising or any outdoor activity. Water belongs in the stomach not the bottle or canteen. So," Drink Up"
6. Avoid coffee, caffeinated drinks, and alcohol that cause increased fluid loss through urination. Avoid them when having fun in the sun.
7. Wear a wet bandana around the neck to help keep body temperature at 98.6 F.
8. Be aware of your special needs. Some medications and herbs increase the sun's effects. If you take antibiotics, diuretics, non-steroidal anti-inflammatories like Ibuprofen, or an herb like St. John's wort, consult with your pharmacists or a certified herbalist.

Sunscreens

1. Sunscreen is usually safe to use when the child is 6-months old.
2. Apply 30 minutes before going outdoors. This gives it time to penetrate the skin. Apply 1-ounce. This will last 2 - 1/2 hours depending on activity. Apply even on cloudy days.
3. "SPF" means Sun Protection Factor
4. SPF 15 = about 4 hours of protection
5. SPF, 30 = about 5 hours of protection
6. Always reapply after swimming or exercising.

Heat Exhaustion

A person can quickly move from exhaustion to the more dangerous heat stroke.

Symptoms:

1. Core body temperature may go from 98.6 F to 105 F
2. Pale clammy skin
3. Profuse sweating
4. Dizziness
5. Weakness
6. Rapid heart rate
7. Vomiting
8. Minor mental confusion
9. Cramps, abdominal and limbs

Treatment:

1. Have the victim lie down in a cool place out of the sun with the legs elevated.
2. Replace fluid loss with water, herbal teas like mint, raspberry or water with sliced lemon or lime.
3. Replace electrolytes, with Rehydration Drink, Vitamin C and mineral-powder packs, and snacks with salt.
4. Wet bandana neck area

Heat Stroke

This is a life-threatening situation. The brain cells are heating up. Call 911 immediately.

Symptoms:

1. Core temperature may be 106 F or higher.
2. Red hot dry skin or may be sweating profusely.
3. Rapid, weak pulse; may be irregular.
4. Low blood pressure.
5. Extreme mental confusion progressing to unconsciousness, brain damage and death.

Treatment:

1. Remove victim from direct sun.
2. Call 911.
3. Undress.
4. Cool temperature rapidly down from 102 to 100 F.

   a. Pour water on victim.
   b. Sponge body with wet towel.
   c. Place cool wet towels on back of neck, chest, under arms, and groin area.
   d. Fan body while wet.
5. Wait 10 minutes after last temperature check and recheck. If temperature starts to climb, start cooling again and recheck every 10 minutes until temperature remains in an acceptable range.
6. If victim is confused or semi-conscious do not give fluids.
   a. If awake and alert give herbal teas, water with lemon or lime.
   b. Give sips every 10 - 15 minutes.
   c. Do not give coffee, back tea, or alcohol.

High Blood Pressure

A blood pressure greater than 140/90 puts a person at risk for heart attack and stroke. If it becomes chronic, kidney damage can occur resulting in the need for dialysis. Seek help from a healthcare professional to normalize your BP.

Prevention:

Most high blood pressures can be controlled through a healthy diet and lifestyle modifications, including stress management, counseling, anger management and daily exercise.

Symptoms:

1. Headache
2. Blurred vision
3. Dizziness

In many cases, it is silent, doing its damage undercover. Therefore, routine physical exams are important and recommended.

Treatment:

1. **A healthcare professional needs to be consulted as early as possible.** If BP is extremely high, stay calm, lie quietly, and have person focus on breathing.
2. Sip a tea made from 3-tsp crushed celery seed. You can add chamomile, catnip, or skullcap herbs to the tea.
3. Hawthorn tea: it dilates the blood vessels allowing normal circulation to occur, therefore reducing pain.
4. If feet and legs are swollen, drink a cup of parsley tea. This will cause urination, taking the fluid load off the heart and thereby reduce the blood pressure.
5. Teas to help lower high blood pressure: celery seed, chamomile, cardamom, fennel, peppermint, green tea.
6. A cup of "non-salty" broth with 1/4 to 1/2 tsp of cayenne pepper and several garlic cloves will help normalize blood pressure. Cayenne pepper increases the force and strength of each heartbeat, dilates capillaries, and takes the load off the heart by increasing circulation to the hands and feet.
7. Some research studies indicate magnesium deficiency may play a role in creating high blood pressure. Daily include green vegetables, mushrooms, beans, whole grains, and purslane (*verdelagas* in Spanish) in your diet.

8. Garlic: along with all its other health-filled qualities, helps normalize blood pressure and reduce cholesterol. As little as 1/2-oz per week will help normalize blood pressure in as few as 14 days. I had one patient, an elder gentleman, who ate 8-cloves a day and normalized his blood pressure. His doctor took him off his blood-pressure medicine. My patient continued with his garlic regime but never told his doctor how he normalized his pressure because he was afraid, he would be laughed at.

Low Blood Pressure

Evaluate. Is there adequate fluid intake? What medications are being taken? Is there a possibility of internal bleeding? Consult with your healthcare professional.

Symptoms:

1. Weak
2. Dizzy
3. May become faint going from sitting to standing.

Treatment:

1. Hydrate with water, add lemon or lime.
2. Rehydration Drink
3. If the person has diabetes, check their blood sugar. If low treat as for hypoglycemia.
4. Ginseng tea on a regular basis can help normalize blood pressure.

Hypothermia

The lowering of body temperature faster than the body can produce heat. This is often caused by sudden emersion of the body into freezing water or being sprayed with cold water, fuel, or other liquids.

Symptoms:

1. Shivering may progress until the violent shakes are uncontrollable and the person is unable to take care of themself.
2. Core temperature falls to 95 to 90 F and the person:
    a. Becomes sluggish.
    b. Irrational
    c. May have a false feeling of warmth.
    d. If the temperature drops further, the result is muscle rigidity, unconsciousness, death.

Treatment:

1. Re-warm the whole body.
    a. Place warm towels on body and cover with blankets.
    b. A warming bath to the torso. (NOTE: Total body emersion should only be done in a hospital setting, because of the increased risk of cardiac arrest and rewarming shock.)
2. Remove wet clothing.
3. Wrap in warmed blankets.

4. Place in warm sleeping bag with another person who is already warm, skin to skin, no clothes. (The individual in the bag with the victim should not stay in the bag too long, or they, too, could become hypothermic.)
5. If the victim is conscious, give them warmed electrolyte drink with honey, or warm cocoa with added sweetener and cayenne.
6. Energy bars with chocolate
7. When the victim is stable, seek medical assistance. There is the danger of rewarming too rapidly and then experiencing "after drop" when the core temperature falls again to unsafe limits.

Indigestion / Gastric Distress

An occasional "sour stomach" is distressing enough, but if ignored it can lead to serious irritation and inflammation to the mucus membranes of the digestive tract. If this occurs on a regular and chronic basis there is cell damage that can lead to cancer.

Prevention:

Following some basic health rules can prevent gastric distress.

1. Slow down. Chew slowly and thoroughly. Gulping and using straws cause a person to swallow air, and what goes in, must go out!
2. Observe your diet. Is it high in carbohydrates? Undigested carbohydrates in the intestines produce gas.
3. Avoid *excessive* consumption of spicy foods, fried foods, fast foods, alcohol, coffee.

4. Eliminate offending foods.
5. Include raw fruits and vegetables in your diet, especially the green "leafies."
6. Avoid large meals at night.
7. Remain sitting up after meals for at least 2 hours.
8. Think pleasant thoughts while eating.

Simple Indigestion

Symptoms:

1. Burning sensation in the chest, especially after eating.
2. Regurgitation of food or sour liquids.
3. Abdominal bloating, gas, cramping.
4. Nausea.

Treatment for Acute Episodes:

1. Teas: ginger, mint, chamomile, fennel, anise
2. Ginger candy for once-in-a-while use only: Add 1 - 2 tsp of ginger in a glass of water. This neutralizes the acid.
3. Adequate liquids: water will dilute the acids.
4. Aloe Vera juice: one ounce daily will soothe and heal the mucus membranes.
5. Licorice tea is antispasmodic and reduces excess production of stomach acid. This is *not* for long term use, or if taking blood pressure medications.

6. Papaya juice and pineapple juice contain enzymes that aid digestion.
7. ***If Digestive Problems Continue See Your Healthcare professional.***

Infected Wounds

The key here is *prevention.* Wash the area and keep it clean. Inspect the wound twice a day.

Symptoms:

1. Redness
2. Swelling
3. Heat
4. Pain
5. Fever
6. Redline or streaks emanating from the wound.
7. Swelling under lymph nodes
8. Bad smell
9. Pus

Leg Cramps

Leg cramps are not necessarily an emergency where you call 911, but it sure does hurt and incapacitate. It is easier to prevent than deal with at two in the morning when it wakes you up.

Prevention:

1. Adequate hydration, especially if active.
2. Daily exercise, to increase circulation and strengthen muscles.
3. Too much caffeine depletes the body of calcium.
4. Are you getting adequate potassium, especially if you are taking a diuretic?
5. Are you getting adequate magnesium in your diet? Add green "leafies."

Treatment:

1. My mom, Dottie, used to get severe leg cramps. She kept a spray bottle with rubbing alcohol and sprayed on her legs when the cramps started.
2. She also used peppermint lotion on her legs and feet.
3. A peppermint tea foot soak increases circulation, done daily it can prevent leg cramps.
4. Placing your bare feet on a cold floor helps.
5. Lift your foot up, leaving the heel on the floor.
6. Use a muscle salve or oil. Salve with black cohosh, cayenne, valerian, willow will help the pain and relax the muscles.
7. Arnica salve to area
8. I've used a heating pad. A hot-water bag works, and the heat helps the leg relax.

9. If cramps increase in frequency contact your physician, there may be an electrolyte imbalance problem, or it may be related to any pharmaceuticals that you are taking.

Lightning Strikes

All thunderstorms are dangerous. Every thunderstorm produces lightening. Dry thunderstorms when are when the rain does not reach the ground, but its lightening does touch down. Up to 75% of people struck by lightning are seriously injured. 70 % have residual effects, and 30 % die. Do not become a statistic. Learn these safety tips.

Safety Tips

The **U.S.** national lightening Safety Institute advises everyone to have their own personal safety plan for when a thunderstorm occurs.

Check The Weather for Your Outside Activity Area and Plan Accordingly.

Indoors:

1. Stay from open windows and doorways.
2. Stay out of bathtubs and hot tubs.
3. Do not use plug in electronics at this time, this could damage computers.
4. Do not use a land line corded phone. Cell phones are safe to use.
5. Do not use ear plugs or headphones, this can lead to ear damage and deafness.

Outdoors: Lightening prefers afternoon so plan your activities accordingly.

1. If working outside, stop and seek shelter. If playing golf, tennis, or any outdoor sport, stop and seek shelter.
2. Avoid hill tops, crests, spires, peaks, and open spaces where you may be the tallest. If there is one tree in a field, do not shelter there. Sit out the storm in a grove of trees, cave, between boulders, under rock ledge, stay close to rock walls. If there is no shelter, crouch.
3. Carrying anything metal can draw lightening to you, golf club, umbrella, hiking sticks, fishing rods.
4. Get out of the water, even if in a small boat.
5. Stay in your vehicle, the metal roof offers good protection.
6. If in a group, spread out so everyone won't be hit at once by a strike.
7. If you feel a tingling in your body, drop to the ground immediately. Lightening is about to strike you. Do not lie flat. Make yourself the smallest target possible. Curl into a ball, head down and arms around your knees, or head between your knees. Hands over your ears.
8. Rubber soled shoes and rubber tires do not protect you from lightening.

Symptoms:

The victim may have been thrown a distance, clothes may be torn or burned. Anything metal on the person may have heated up, causing burns. The victim is usually confused and may be temporarily blind or deaf. Amnesia is common and usually transient.

The person may stop breathing for up to 30 minutes and then start breathing again. The head, neck, and shoulders are the parts of the body usually affected. In severe cases there may be fernlike patterns of burns over the skin.

Treatment:

1. Maintain an airway, assist breathing if needed.
2. Cardiac arrest can occur, start CPR.
3. Assume the victim has been thrown by the impact. Immobilize the spine, especially the cervical (neck) spine. A clear or red-tinged fluid from the ear may indicate cerebral spinal leak.
4. There may be muscle contractions, tremors, and seizures. (See Seizures)
5. See burns.
6. Examine the victim for any other injuries and treat accordingly.
7. Keep the victim warm, out of the elements, and insulate from the ground.

It is imperative to transport the patient to a medical facility as soon as possible. As soon as there is cell service call 911.

There are residual effects, brain, neuropsychiatric symptoms, vision, and hearing issues. These usually develop slowly over time, and because of the delay, lightening as a cause can often be overlooked as a cause of symptoms. Keep in contact with your healthcare professional.

Morning Sickness

There are only a few plants that are safe for the unborn child. There are fewer pharmaceutical drugs that are safe. Be very careful of what goes into the developing baby. The remedies given here are proven safe.

Symptoms:

Nausea upon awaking, sometimes throughout the day when you are pregnant.

Treatment:

1. Ginger tea, ginger candy, throughout the day as needed.
2. Soda crackers, sometimes helps if eaten when first wake up.
3. One tsp of bee pollen in fruit juice daily, B complex vitamins will help but a pill may be too strong, bee pollen is gentler and contains other nutrients plus digestive enzymes.
4. Raspberry tea.
5. Eat a snack an hour before you go to bed.
6. Spearmint tea, peppermint tea are safe if taken in moderate amounts.
    a. Large amounts could trigger miscarriage, especially if there is a history of miscarriage.
    b. One cup a day as needed.
    c. May sip throughout the day.

Natural Protection From Toxins

Antioxidant Enzymes:

1. **Superoxide Dismutase**: The first line of defense that the body has against superoxide free radicals. Considered the most effective antioxidant.
2. **Catalase**: Removes hydrogen peroxide molecules, which are the byproducts of reactions created by SOD.
3. **Glutathione Peroxidase**: Consists of the amino acid glutathione and trace mineral selenium. Its focus is the free radicals called peroxides, prevents destruction of cell membranes.
4. **Symptoms of Excess Peroxide Free Radicals**:
    a. Heart disease,
    b. Liver disease
    c. Premature aging
    d. Skin cancer
    e. Age spots
    f. Dermatitis
    g. Psoriasis
5. **Methionine Reductase**: Effective against the free radical called hydroxyl radical. This is commonly formed through reactions involving heavy metals and can damage any type of organic cellular tissue. They are the main toxins generated by:
    a. Exposure to excessive radiation

b. Can be created when we burn fat molecules to produce energy, as in strenuous exercise or dieting.

6. B-Complex Vitamins: Rids excess metals from the intestine tract. Supports nerves. **Source**: Bee Pollen, Bee Propolis

7. **Bioflavonoids and Vitamin C**: Improve immune system, counteracts radiation, antioxidant, facilitates absorption of iron, protects against lead, mercury, DDT, cadmium: **Source**:

   a. Citrus fruits

   b. Broccoli

   c. Green peppers,

   d. Strawberries

   e. Tomatoes

   f. Red chili

   g. Parsley

   h. Cilantro

   i. Cantaloupe

8. **Calcium**: Binds with aluminum, cadmium, fluoride, mercury and other toxins. Decreases absorption of strontium 90, calcium 45, and other radioisotopes. **Source**:

   a. Sesame seeds

   b. Almonds

   c. Soybeans

   d. Soy products

   e. Sea veggies

f. Mallow

g. Comfrey

h. Bone set

i. Cinnamon

9. **Chaparral**: Contains Nordihydroguaiaretic acid, an anti-tumor agent, stabilizes Vitamin A, denies tumor food, antioxidant.

10. **Chlorophyll** (similar in structure to hemoglobin) : Decreases radiation toxicity, detoxes lead, heightens efficiency of all the tissues and organs, nerves, heart contractions stronger, diastolic period longer, helps lower BP, helps in constipation, encourages peristaltic action of intestines, helps protect wound infections because of magnesium, increases new cell granulations, dries wounds, limits secretions, regulates acidity of gastric juices, detox lead. **Source**:

    a. Nettles

    b. Parsley

    c. Cilantro

    d. Broccoli

    e. Blue green algae.

11. **Fermented Foods**: Produces friendly bacteria which promotes digestion, counteracts toxins, builds immune system, detoxifies the body. **Source**:

    a. Miso

    b. Tempeh

c. Tamari

d. Sauerkraut

e. Yogurt

f. Kefir

g. "Pickled foods"

12. **Garlic**: Protects from free radicals, suppress synthesis of LDH, lowers cholesterol reduces lipoproteins, anthelmintics (worms), excreted thru lungs and skin, cleans out heavy metals, especially lead.

13. **Ginko**: antioxidant, increases oxygen.

14. **Ginseng**: antioxidant, enhances energy.

Near-Drowning

Drowning is the 2nd leading cause of accidental death in the US. Most of these deaths could have been avoided. First and foremost, learn to swim and make sure your children know how to swim. My mother, Dottie, didn't know how to swim as a child and as an adult nearly drowned in a swimming pool. She made sure I had swimming lessons and knew how to take care of myself in the water.

Basic rules of water safety:

1. Learn to swim and be sure all family members can swim.
2. If you have a boat, backyard pool, live near water, take a course in basic rescue and water safety.
3. Never swim alone, never leave a child alone near a pool, even for a second.

4. Make sure a place is safe before you swim., depth, rock, tree debris, etc.
5. Don't dive into unknown or shallow water.
6. Know your limitations.
7. Get out of the water at the first sign of a storm or rising waves.
8. If there is a pool on your property, safety is YOUR responsibility. There are 4 main causes of pool accidents:
    a. Inability to swim
    b. Inadequate barriers
    c. Lack of supervision
    d. Intoxicants, both legal and illegal substances
9. Alcohol and other intoxicants and water sports **DO NOT MIX**
10. If you are caught in a riptide, swim to shore at a 45' angle to the shore. Swimming directly to shore will cause you to be pulled out to sea.
11. If you are thrown overboard and are not wearing a life jacket:
    a. Try to remove your pants, and shoes, especially heavy boots.
    b. Knot the leg ends and swirl them over your head to fill them with air.
    c. Roll the waist shut, put the pants under water, rest head between inflated legs.
    d. I have never had to do this, but if you don't panic, it could save your life.

12. Use HELP, the Heat Escape Lessening Position.
    a. If wearing a life jacket, cross arms and place hands on shoulders or neck.
    b. Cross ankles.
    c. Bring knees to chest.
    d. Practice this before you need it.
13. Know what to do in emergencies, stay calm!
14. Always watch children. Teach them:
    a. Never push anyone into the water, or to duck someone's head underwater.
    b. Always **walk** around pools or docks.
    c. Do not go down a waterslide headfirst or sideways.
15. Boats and docks, put ins and take outs are not playgrounds.
16. Teach them NEVER to cry "Help" unless there is a real reason. Remember the story about the little boy who cried wolf?
17. Keep rescue equipment by the pool and in the boat.
18. Remove all toys from the pool or boat after use so children aren't tempted to reach for them.

Signs That Someone is in Trouble:

1. Thrashing arms
2. Bobbing up or down
3. Head tilted back, mouth open, often a drowning person can't yell for help.

4. If you are not trained, do not swim to the victim.
5. When the person is out of reach, use a long branch, a paddle, a towel, or pants, anything that may help.
6. You can make a buoy using a plastic jug with a rope tied on the handle, even throwing (an underhanded throw) a plastic cooler will help, giving the person something to grab hold of and help them stay afloat.
7. If you are in a boat, extend a paddle, pull them to the boat and tow them ashore.
8. Respect the water and have fun!

Near Drowning:

1. If the victim is not breathing begin mouth to mouth respirations.
2. Call 911.
3. If there is no pulse, begin chest compressions.
4. Suspect neck injuries.
5. Do not move victim.
6. Give First Aid for shock.
7. Hypothermia may be a factor. Gently remove wet clothes and cover with blankets.
8. Even if a victim says they feel fine they need to be evaluated by a physician.
9. With signs of respiratory distress seek medical help immediately. You already called 911, right?

Herbal Support:

Use herbs that soothe the respiratory tract, prevents coughing and expels mucus or foreign material. The goal is to prevent severe coughing episodes that may trigger laryngeal spasms causing acute swelling that can restrict respirations causing suffocation that leads to death. At the first symptoms of distress:

Symptoms Of Respiratory Distress:

1. Coughing increases
2. Audible wheezing with breathing
3. Increased pain with breathing or coughing
4. Rapid respirations

5. Rapid pulse
6. Difficulty breathing, straining to breathe.
7. Breathlessness, breathing comes with gasps.
8. Gurgling sounds in the chest
9. Cyanosis: first signs, lips, and nail beds blue

Herbal Remedies:

1. **Elderberry tincture**, lozengier or dried herb as tea, 15 to thirty drops of the tincture, will help lower fever.
2. **Thyme tea**, add juice of 1 lemon and 1 tablespoon of honey. Drink 2 to 3 times a day to control coughing.
3. **Licorice tea** soothes mucus membranes, decreases swelling that can lead to respiratory difficulty. This is for short term use only, 1 cup, 2 - 3 times a day.
4. **Slippery elm** tea or lozenges soothes the respiratory tract.
5. **Anise tea** for cough, and expelling phlegm
6. **Marshmallow, Yerba Negrita**: make a tea of roots to sooth and calm a sore throat and respiratory tract.
7. **Mullein leaf tea** soothes and acts as an expectorant. Strain the tea to remove the tiny hairs that are on the leaf and that may cause additional irritation. Adding mint or chamomile or honey will improve the taste.
8. **Grindelia tea** as expectorant, add honey as this is bitter.
9. **Bee pollen** will support loss of B-complex Vitamins that occurs during stress.
10. **Ginseng tea** supplies nutrients to a stressed body

11. **Chamomile tea** will calm and relax the near drowning victim.
12. **Osha root tea** can prevent lung infections.
13. **Foods high in Vitamin A** enhance the immune system and protects the lungs (those yellow vegetables and fruits).
14. **Rehydration Drink** will provide electrolyte replacement and electrolyte balance.

Overdose Of Medication

Pharmaceuticals, Prescription Drugs, Over the counter medications, Illegal drugs

An overdose is not poisoning. It can happen accidentally, by unintentionally taking too many pills, or as a direct intention to commit suicide. Most overdoses are accidental and can lead to permanent damage to the body and mind. In 2022, 109,000 Americans died of drug overdose, up from 70,237 in 2017. Opioids were involved in many of those deaths. Opioids are psychoactive chemicals similar to the synthetic drug morphine. They kill more than 136 people every day.

Prevention:

All prescription medications should be in a locked cupboard or locked box. Supplements and vitamins must be out of the reach of children.

Doctors, Physician Assistants, and Nurse Practitioners can familiarize themselves with alternative treatments and remedies, such as acupuncture, chiropractic, naprapathy, physical therapy, massage, and external remedies such as salves, ointments, and patches such as Tiger Balm, Lidocaine, roll-on muscle relievers, and psychotherapy to name a few. There are herbal pain and anxiety and depression relievers. Psychospiritual issues are often buried and express themselves as somatic complaints. Anxiety tenses muscles causing pain. In the holistic approach the whole person is treated.

Symptoms:

1. Drifting in and out of consciousness
2. Pupils smaller, becoming pinpoint.
3. Slow breaths,4 - 6 a minute
4. Blue lips
5. Blue fingernails

Treatment:

There are no herbal remedies for an overdose. Seek help immediately!

1. If someone you know is taking heroin or you suspect the overuse of a pain medication, Naloxone (Narcan) kits are now being made available to the general public.
2. Get one and learn how to use it.
3. If the person is unconscious, barely breathing, intravenous Naloxone must be given.
4. The person needs medical help immediately.
5. If brain damage has not occurred, the person will "come out of it ". However, the danger is not over.
6. Naloxone has a short life in the body.
7. The drug ingested may have a longer life and a "relapse "may occur.

If left alone or not taken to a medical facility where they can be monitored and treated if a relapse does occur, they can die.

Pain

There are two kinds of pain, acute and chronic. Chronic pain persists for weeks and months. What we are discussing here is acute pain.

Acute pain

1. Give your pain a number, 1 the least, and 10 the most. The goal is to not get a number over 5.
2. Over 5 is harder to control and may take longer to control.
3. Do pain therapy when your pain is about 5.
4. What type of pain do you have? burning, sharp, stabbing?
5. Does it come and go or is it constant?
6. Does it occur with movement?
7. These would be important things to mention to your healthcare professional.

Treatment:

1. **Clove oil** for tooth ache: apply directly to gum around tooth.
2. **Turmeric**: for arthritis pain, take 1 - 2 capsules several times a day or sprinkle daily on food.
3. **Rosemary tea**
4. **Peppermint or lavender** oil or salve externally
5. **Hot pack** alternating with cold packs for 15 minutes to painful aches and sprains, apply as often as needed.

6. **Cayenne** in a poultice or in salve applied to area. It blocks the pain signals that come from the nerves just under the skin and prevents nerve cells from making more pain signal cells for up to 8 hours.
7. **Drink a cup of dill**, chamomile, or lavender tea when the cramps of colic begin.
8. **Willow or Aspen**, or Cottonwood made into a salve with cayenne will help achy joints and muscles.
9. **Rest**: lie quietly, observe your breathing, with each breathe exhale out pain, relax each part of your body, inhale healing energy. A tense body affects every part of the body, the nerves. The tightened muscles increase the pain.
10. **Valerian** Tea: Relaxing teas and tinctures like Valerian will relax the muscle. (It does really taste like old dirty socks, quite an acquired taste, but it works on most people.)
11. **Catnip** is a muscle relaxant.
12. **Hot bath** with Epsom salts, add lavender, sink deep into your water, breathe out and visualize yourself floating on a South Sea lagoon.
13. **If the pain is related to a wound**, severe injury, or the abdomen, see your healthcare professional.

Poisoning

Poisoning is an injury due to swallowing, inhaling, touching, or by injecting certain chemicals, gases, or venoms. Some are poisonous only in higher dosages than recommended. Children are especially vulnerable to even small amounts of substances.

How you treat depends on:

1. The symptoms
2. Age of victim
3. What substance has caused the poisoning?

Prevention:

1. If you have young children, grandchildren, great grandchildren, or will have visitors with young children, don't wait until an incident occurs to have the Poison Control Center (PCC) number by your landline or in your cell phone. Post it on your refrigerator where it can easily be seen among all the other magnets decorating the refrigerator door. The national toll-free poison emergency number: 800 222 1222.
2. Keep any potential toxic products locked away from curious eyes and hands, this includes medications and vitamin supplements.
3. Use natural, non-toxic products. The appendix has safe and effective recipes you can make yourself and save money.
4. If you are in a remote cabin without cell service and there is a twisty-turny washboard road, have a plan before an incident occurs. Gasoline and kerosene MUST be in a locked place. Show the containers to your children and teach them that they are poison and can cause serious consequences if they play with them.
5. Keep your cell phone charged. In remote areas use a solar charger.
6. Be alert for clues: empty pill bottles, or containers. An unconscious person may have stains on them or their clothes or have an unusual odor on their breath.

Symptoms:

1. Burns or redness around the mouth and lips
2. Chemical smell to the breath (think paint thinners, gasoline)
3. Vomiting
4. Difficulty breathing, no breathing
5. Drowsiness
6. Unconsciousness
7. Confusion, altered mental state
8. Restlessness, agitation
9. Seizures

Even if symptoms are minor or absent but you suspect poisoning, call the Poison Control and 911 and have the person transported to the closest Emergency Room. Do not give anything until told to do so by the Poison Control Center.

Swallowed Poison:

Do not induce vomiting if you have reason to believe the person has taken a substance that will burn or damage the mucus membranes of the mouth, throat, or esophagus. These may be acid or alkaline, household cleaners, kerosene, gasoline, pesticides, herbicides.

In 1993 the PCC advised giving syrup of ipecac to induce vomiting in the victim. Since vomiting removes only half or less of the poison, the PCC also advised using activated charcoal to remove the poison. In 2019 there is controversy regarding the use of syrup of ipecac. The American Academy of Pediatrics no longer advises the use of ipecac. The American Association of Poison Control

Centers still maintains that the syrup does have a place in the treatment of poisoning. They recommend letting the local ER decide what is the best treatment. There is a danger of aspiration, fluid getting into the lung.

In the pre-hospital situation, evaluate the situation:

1. What are the symptoms?
2. What was swallowed?
3. How far is it to the nearest emergency center?
4. Keep calm and then make your decision.

Treatment:

1. **Ipecac**: No longer can be bought over the counter. Ask the pharmacist or order on the internet.
    a. Usual dosage: Two tablespoons or 1/2 ounce of syrup followed by two 8-ounce glasses of water.
    b. This is an adult dose.
    c. The PCC will give correct dose for a child, follow directions on the label. If no vomiting occurs, repeat in 20 minutes.

Precautions:

d. Do not give if drowsy or unconscious, or if have swallowed corrosive substance or gasoline or kerosene.

e. Do Not Give if pregnant, it causes uterine contractions that may lead to miscarriage.

f. Do not make your own, the fluid extract is 14 times stronger than the syrup and can cause heart toxicity and death.

2. On the trail and someone has eaten some mushrooms or a plant that is poison, induce gagging by placing a spoon or other such object gently on the back of the throat. It is wise to stand on the side of a person when doing this. It is unwise to place your finger there.

3. If you have no ipecac and you are home or at base camp these suggestions may be of value:

   Place the products below in a half liter of water and give the awake, alert person to drink:

   a. 2 tablespoons of mild soap

   b. 2 tablespoons dried mustard

   c. Have the person drink another 1/2 liter of water to dilute the poison. Water is a great diuretic (makes a person pee) and the poison is flushed from the body.

4. Activated charcoal:

   a. Comes as a powder, liquid, tablet, or capsule.

   b. The charcoal binds with the poison and prevents it from being absorbed. It will not bind with a corrosive agent or petroleum products.

   c. **Dosage**: Shake the liquid for at least 30 seconds.

   d. Mix the powder with water to the consistency of a milk shake.

   e. Have the victim drink it.

f. Follow with water to flush out and prevent constipation. The poison will be reabsorbed if not removed in a bowel movement.

5. White or green clay absorbs and eliminates the poison in bowel movement:

    a. **Dosage**:

    b. 1 teaspoon in 8 ounces of water,

    c. Followed by a 8 ounce glass of water.

    d. Without water, the poison will be reabsorbed, and constipation occurs adding to an already distressed condition.

Poisoning on the Skin

This can occur with dry or wet chemicals. With all chemicals, use gloves to remove contaminated clothing. If no gloves are available, use tongs or other tong-like objects. Dispose of gloves and clothing as you would any hazardous material.

Treatment:

1. Wet substance:

    a. Flood the skin with a constant stream of water for 15 to 30 minutes.

    b. After flooding wash gently with mild soap and water.

2. Dry powder like substance:

    a. Brush off the skin being careful not to get into eyes or to inhale into the lungs.

b. Cover your mouth and the victim's mouth with a bandanna or scarf.

c. Do not add water as this may activate the chemical.

3. Call the PCC for further instructions.

Poison in the Eye

Call for help immediately. The person must go to the local emergency center immediately. Vision is precious, don't waste time.

Treatment:

1. Gently flush the eye with cool or lukewarm water for 20 minutes or while waiting for EMS to arrive.
2. You can use a kitchen baster, bulb syringe or gently pour using a cup.
3. Be careful not to get rinse fluid on other parts of the body.

Inhaled Poison:

After making sure the person is safe call 911.

Rescuer:

1. Do not breathe toxic fumes.
2. Cover mouth and nose with wet bandana, scarf, or cloth.
3. If these are not available, take two deep breaths of fresh air and hold your breath.

Treatment:

1. Get the person to fresh air immediately.
2. Open doors and windows.

3. Place victim in rescue position on the left side, loosen clothing, keep comfortable.
4. Access airway and breathing.
5. If necessary, start rescue breathing and CPR.
6. Even if the victim seems fine and refuses to go to the ER, seek help immediately. It could take a while for symptoms to appear.

Symptoms:

1. Bluish lips
2. Unusual breath odor
3. Chest pain, chest tightness, shortness of breath, difficulty breathing, coughing
4. Dizziness
5. Headache
6. Drowsiness
7. Heart palpitations
8. Irritability
9. Loss of bladder control
10. Muscle twitching
11. Seizures
12. Nausea and vomiting
13. Weakness

Ingestion of Button Batteries

These are the small flat batteries used in watches and other electronics. A battery can burn the mucus membranes in as little as two hours. If you suspect a child has swallowed one of these, go immediately to an emergency center. It must be removed by a physician.

Ingestion of Medical Patches

Carefully inspect the child's roof of their mouth. The patches often lodge there. Call ER before you go, then they can be prepared for your arrival with the proper equipment.

Post Emergency Treatments:

Ingestion:

1. **Chamomile tea** to calm the victim and family, drink as needed.
2. **Milk Thistle**: Traditionally used to protect and regenerate the liver after toxic ingestions, esp. after intense alcohol use, and mushroom poisoning. Use the tincture as it is poorly absorbed from the digestive tract.

   Dosage: 15 – 25 drops, 4 - 5 times daily
3. **Dandelion root tea**: Can be found in most yards if not poisoned by those wanting a monoculture lawn. Heals and restores liver function.

   Dosage: 2 - 3 cups daily, is also a diuretic and helps eliminate some poisons.
4. **Burdock root tea** neutralizes any remaining poison.

Dosage 1 cup, 2 - 3 times daily for 2 -3 days.

5. **Slippery Elm tea** or throat lozenges for throat irritations, after ingestion or vomiting.
6. **Fenugreek seed, licorice** (not for use if pregnant) mullein leaf, yerba negrita, calendula are teas for irritated throat.
7. **Aloe Vera** for throat: Dosage: 1 ounce 2 - 3 times a day
8. **Mint or Lavender tea** for nausea and calming, as needed.
9. **Green tea, rose petal tea, mint tea** for inflammation: The whole body may "feel on fire."
10. **B-complex** for stress and healing nerves, bee pollen or pill.
11. **Vitamin C,** 1000mg -3000mg as an antioxidant, and to prevent infections.

Skin

1. **Aloe Vera**: gel or leaf applied to irritated area, several times a day as needed.
2. **Calendula,** comfrey, lavender, rose petal: salve, lotion, poultice to the irritated skin.
3. **Olive oil**: liquid or salve is soothing and repairs damaged skin.
4. **Cucumber**, fresh, organic: juice or place in water for 1 - 2 hours. Strain, use soft cloth, dip in liquid, place on irritated skin.
5. **Plantain**: usually found in yards unless a monocrop of grass exists. Salve, lotion or juice from fresh leaf, place on area.

6. **Zinc 50 – 60 mg.** a day helps to repair the skin; zinc ointment may be used externally.

Acute Reaction to Environmental Toxins

Acute reactions can happen anywhere or any time. There are many chemicals in our environment. It could be said we are a chemical generation. We encounter chemicals by breathing, touching, and ingesting. Our bodies react to even small particles of chemicals or radiation. Chronic exposure can lead to cancers and neurological breakdowns. Often, we may not know what the chemical or agent might be. Acute responses and symptoms are varied. It depends on the chemical and the person. I have listed some common reactions.

Symptoms:

1. Chest becomes tight.
2. Difficulty getting your breath.
3. Audible chest wheezes or dry wheezy cough.
4. Headache that gets progressively worse.
5. Irritated, watery eyes.
6. Runny nose.
7. Nausea and vomiting.
8. Rashes
9. Neurological symptoms, tremors, severe shaking, seizures asthma attacks, progressing to respiratory collapse.

Seizure

A seizure or convulsion is usually an attack of unconsciousness preceded by tonic / clonic (jerking) muscle contractions of a violent nature. However, there are milder forms that may only be brief, momentary loss of contact with the surroundings. They can occur with someone who has epilepsy or be the result of infection, high fever, or associated with head injury, brain, or nervous-system disorders.

Symptoms:

1. Rigidity of body muscles, usually lasting from a few seconds to perhaps a minute. This is followed by jerking movements.
2. The victim may stop breathing.
3. Bluish discoloration of the face and lips
4. May bite tongue
5. Foaming at the mouth or drooling
6. Loss of bladder and bowel control

Treatment:

1. Prevent the victim from hurting themselves.
2. Do not restrain or hold down.
3. Do not place a blunt object into the mouth.
4. Do not pour liquids into the mouth.
5. Do not place a child in a tub of water.
6. Give artificial respiration if indicated.

7. When the seizure has subsided, place the person on their side, turn head to one side, to allow secretions to drain and prevent choking.

8. Cover and keep warm.

Call for medical help if seizures persist without stopping, any injuries occur, or if the person continues in a state of confusion.

Shock

Shock is life-threatening. There are many causes: large burns, major blood loss, dehydration, severe allergic reactions, and heavy bleeding inside the body.

Symptoms:

1. Weak rapid pulse
2. Cold sweat
3. Pale cold, clammy skin
4. Blood pressure low
5. Weakness
6. Mental confusion

Treatment:

1. Have the person lie down, the feet a little higher than the head.
2. Cover with a blanket.
3. Stop any bleeding.
4. If conscious give the electrolyte drink "Rehydration."

5. Seek medical help immediately.

Splinter, Slivers, Cactus Spines

Don't ignore. They can become infected. If you have diabetes, don't attempt self-remedy, see your primary care doctor.

Treatment:

1. Wash the area with mild soap and water. If the water source is questionable, boil the water and let it cool.
2. Try to pull out with tweezers.
3. If just under the skin, sterilize a needle by heating the point in a clear point of a flame for several minutes. Allow it to cool and *ease* the splinter out.
4. Don't dig deep with unsterile implements.
5. Use a white bread poultice.
6. If the splinter is glass or is embedded deeply, a medical person should be seen.
7. To draw the splinter out, I keep a jar of pinesap in my cupboard. I soften the pinesap and place it over area and secure it with a Band-Aid.
8. Cactus removal: when walking or hiking in the desert be especially careful where you put your hands and feet. Jumping chollas do jump!
    a. If a piece of cactus is attached to your skin, pantleg or sock, knock it off with a comb, a stick or piece of wood.
    b. Large stickers or spines can be removed with tweezers.

c. Wash the area with soap and water and apply an antibiotic salve, preferably an herbal antibiotic salve.

d. Keep clean

e. Observe for signs of infection and treat.

f. If you have diabetes and your blood sugar is elevated it may be a sign of an infection. See your medical practitioner.

Sprains

A sprain occurs when you twist, turn, stretch, or roll a joint beyond its normal range. The ligaments that are overstretched may tear. Ankle sprains are the most common injuries is the USA. Without proper treatment you could face lifelong chronic foot and ankle problems.

Symptoms:

1. Swelling
2. Pain
3. Decreased movement, cannot move
4. Limited use of joint
5. Numbness
6. Skin pale or bluish, feels cool to touch.
7. If you hear a crunching sound on movement, there may be a fracture.

If a sprain doesn't improve after 72 hours of home treatment, see a medical professional.

CAUTION: ***bruises may be immediate, take hours or even days to appear***. If you have osteoporosis, diabetes, nerve damage to feet or legs, or are taking blood thinners (baby aspirin is *not* for babies. It is 81 mg. It is a strong blood thinner, or it would not have been prescribed). **Seek professional help immediately.**

Treatment:

Depending on the severity of the sprain, or if it is an ankle sprain, you will be at rest for 1 - 3 weeks. Your health care practitioner will determine the best schedule for you. **REMEMBER**: the choice is up to you: adhere to the recommended rest period or cope with chronic pain, a decrease in activity, and an increase in money spent to control symptoms.

It's always better to prevent injury. The American Academy of Orthopedics recommends exercising strengthen muscles and balance to prevent falls.

1. You don't have to buy this **RICE**, (Rest Ice Compression Elevate) just remember to use it.
    a. **REST** ankle.
    b. **ICE**: do this immediately to keep swelling down.
        - wrap ice in towel or washcloth,
        - No ice? Use a cold-water compress.
        - Apply to area, leave on for 15 minutes.
        - Do this 4 times a day.
        - If you are diabetic or have nerve or blood vessel damage, use cold-water compress, and remove after 5 minutes.

c. **COMPRESSION**:

- Use an elastic wrap on ankle to support it and relieve swelling.
- Do not wrap too tightly.
- Do not go to bed with the compression wrap on.

d. **ELEVATE** foot to a level above your heart to reduce swelling.

2. Anti-inflammatory:

   a. Turmeric, basil, black pepper, cumin, and ginger can be added to food, and eaten throughout the day.

   b. Ginger tea and green tea taste great and are stronger when used together. One can also take turmeric in capsules.

   c. Aspen, Cottonwood, and Willow are pain relievers and anti-inflammatory, can be taken as tea or tincture.

3. Compress of apple cider vinegar will help sore muscles; do this 2 - 3 times a day, before or after an icing.
4. Apply arnica salve or liniment to area. Take arnica homeopathic as directed.
5. For pain relief, see **PAIN.**
6. Splint as you would a fracture.
7. Check pulses, skin temperature and color every 15 minutes if in a splint. Loosen as needed.
8. If it is necessary to walk, make or find material for a crutch. Do not put weight on the injured area.

What is the most important therapy? Rest!

Stroke

A stroke usually involves a clot in a blood vessel to the brain or a rupture of a blood vessel in the brain. Prompt medical attention is necessary.

Symptoms:

1. Paralysis or weakness on one side of the body
2. Difficulty breathing and swallowing.
3. Slurred speech or unable to talk.
4. One side of the mouth droops. Ask the person to smile if you think they may have had a stroke; if one side of the mouth droops that is an indication.
5. Pupils unequal in size
6. Loss of bladder and bowl control
7. Headache
8. Confusion
9. Slight dizziness, ringing in the ears.
10. Memory changes
11. Disturbance in the normal personality
12. Unconsciousness

First Aid

1. Protect the patient from accidents. Position on side, head to one side.
2. Cover with blanket.
3. Loosen clothing.

4. Maintain open airway.
5. Begin artificial respiration if not breathing. CPR if no pulse.
6. Do not give fluids even if the person is conscious, the throat muscles may be paralyzed, allowing the liquid to go into the lungs.
7. Call for medical help immediately. Do not attempt to drive them yourself. You can't drive and give CPR at the same time.

Sunburn

This is usually a minor burn that affects the outer layer of skin. Depending on the circumstances it can usually be treated at home.

Symptoms:

1. Bright red skin
2. Painful
3. Small blisters may occur.

Treatment:

1. Cold apple cider vinegar compresses.
2. Olive oil soothes.
3. Aloe vera; commercial gel or leaf that is split open.
4. Fresh cucumber juice soothes and takes away the heat. Can't juice? apply thin slices.
5. Comfrey, lavender salves, soothes and heals.
6. Fresh, unsweetened yoghurt to area.

7. Chamomile tea helps to relax.

Toothache

Why does it always happen in the middle of the night?

Treatment:

1. Cloves
   a. Chew on a few pieces of dried cloves, place next to painful tooth.
   b. Make a strong clove tea, dip a small piece of cotton into the tea and place on the tooth where the pain is.
   c. Clove oil on a piece of cotton and place on tooth; use a cotton swab to place the oil.
2. Echinacea root can be used the same way. One of its nick names is "Toothache plant." If you have a tincture, place some on the cotton and place around tooth.
3. Make that appointment to see the dentist that you have been putting off for a while!

TIPS ON "HOW TO DO IT"

I have included some basics, such as how to boil water, as some who read this book may be novices in the kitchen. We all must start somewhere. But don't wait for an emergency. Become familiar with these before the need arises so you will be calm and competent.

Aloe Vera Gel

1. Choose a full plump leaf.
2. On a cutting board with a sharp knife, slice it from the mother plant.
3. Peel back the tough outer skin and scoop out the gel.

Apply directly where needed.

Boil Water

Drinking water must be protected from contamination, especially from the feces of animals and humans. Contaminated water is often the cause of diarrhea, which can be fatal in babies and the elderly.

It is best to keep a supply of purified water on hand to use in emergencies or disaster situations. If you suspect your water has become contaminated, don't even use it to brush your teeth. Boiling water kills bacteria, viruses, and parasites. Boiling water is more effective water-purification than treating it with chlorine bleach or other chemicals. The best type of containers to store water in are BPA-free plastic or glass containers that have tight-fitting screw caps. The containers should be disinfected before filling them with purified water. You can either do this by using bleach or pour boiling water into the container. Do not boil plastic containers. To use bleach: add 1 TBSP of liquid bleach to one gallon of water; pour into the container to be disinfected; let it set for 10 minutes; pour out the solution; rinse with purified water; pour out the rinse water. Replace with the purified water. Cap. The water must be used within six months.

To boil containers for disinfecting: in a large pan, submerge the glass container; bring to a rolling boil then boil for 10 minutes.

Boiled Water:

Water boils at 212 °F at sea level. The higher the altitude, the lower the atmospheric pressure. The less atmospheric pressure, the easier it is for water molecules to escape into the air. Water comes to a boil quicker at higher altitudes. The boiling point of water is higher on a stormy day and will take longer to come to a boil. Choose a pot that's large enough to hold the water you want to boil. A short wide pan will come to boiling point sooner than a tall narrow one.

Boiling Water:

1. Use cold water.
2. Don't fill the pot all the way up; boiling water increases in volume.
3. Put on stove or campfire or hot coals.
4. Placing a lid on the pan can speed the process.
5. When you see steam coming out of the lid, carefully lift the lid and look.

6. Bubbles indicate water is boiling; wait for the bubbles to rise to the top of the pot.
7. Slow boil: 205 °F, noticeable movement with large bubbles.
8. Rolling boil: 212 °F, the water is rolling, vigorously bubbling, and steaming.

If you are purifying water, it must boil for 10 minutes.

Measuring Temperatures:

FAHRENHEIT		CELSIUS/CENTIGRADE
32 °F water freezes	=	0 °C
115 °F water simmers	=	46 °C
130 °F water scalds	=	54 °C
212 °F water boils	=	100 °C

Compresses

A compress is an external application that is usually dipped into an herbal solution or vinegar used to treat superficial ailments, stimulate circulation of blood or lymph, relieve colic and muscle spasms, reduce inflammation, reduce fevers, and restore vitality. Two rules to remember: 1) If the affected area is red and hot, apply warm moist compresses. 2) If the affected area itches and oozes clear fluid, use cold wet compresses.

1. Boil water and allow it to cool to 100°F to 108°F.
2. Make an herbal tea, use plain water or vinegar.
3. Dip a towel or cloth into the water or strained tea.

4. Squeeze out the extra liquid.
5. Apply as hot as can be tolerated, but no more than 115°F.
6. Cover with a dry flannel cloth, or sheet of thin plastic wrap.
7. When it begins to cool, apply another warm compress, and repeat the process.

Cough Syrup

Syrup is used for coughs, throat inflammations, and to soothe the stomach and intestinal tract. Syrup can be made with honey or sugar. Natural, local, unprocessed, and unheated honey is the best choice. **CAUTION: Honey is not given to infants or children under 1 year of age.** I have included both honey and sugar recipes. Use raw organic sugar if available. It is a wise idea to make these up in advance and be prepared.

Preparation of Honey Syrup:

1. Two ounces of herbs (See Herbs) added to
2. One quart water
3. Boil gently to reduce to 1 pint.
4. Strain
5. While still warm add 2 to 4 ounces of honey

Making A Stronger Syrup:

1. One gallon honey
2. Four cups total herbs
3. Tie in a cheesecloth
4. Bring to boil.

5. Turn down to a simmer for one hour, may be thinned with purified water if too thick.

Simple Sugar Syrup:

1. Place 14 ounces sugar into blender.
2. Add 14 ounces of water and blend on high for 3 to 4 minutes.
3. Add another 8 ounces water and blend another 1 to 2 minutes.
4. Add another 14 ounces of sugar and blend.
5. Simple syrup is safe for children under 1 year.

Herbal Baths

There are baths for every purpose and several ways to prepare your bath.

1. Tie a handful or about 1/2 cup of herbs in cheesecloth or washcloth.
2. Place the cloth in a cotton muslin bag or large rice-cooking ball, and place in the tub under the running water.
3. Place the herbs in a covered nonmetal pot, cover with water.
4. Bring to a boil and simmer covered for 10 - 20 minutes.
5. Strain the material and pour the liquid into your tub.
6. Soak for at least 20 minutes.
7. Enjoy, relax, and don't forget to compost the plant material.

Mustard Plaster

This is a well-known folk remedy that has been used for hundreds of years. Placed on the chest, it breaks up congestion, relieves asthma, bronchial pneumonia, and pleurisy, and eliminates coughs, head colds and flu. It can be used to treat sprains and painful joints. Mustard seeds, *Sinapis alba*, are rubefacients, bringing circulation to the skin and thereby bringing heat, nutrition, and oxygen.

***CAUTION**: The actual paste NEVER comes into direct contact with the skin.* If left on too long, it can blister the skin. Do not put it on sensitive places. Mustard plasters should not be used on children under 6 years.

1. Mix 4 TBSP flour and 1 TBSP of powdered mustard seed (if using wild mustard seed, use 2 TBSP seeds). Now is the time to use your mortar and pestle.
2. Mix with enough cold water to make a thick paste.
3. Spread paste on cotton, flannel, or hemp cloth.
4. Place a thin cloth on the skin.
5. Place mustard cloth on top of the thin cloth.
6. Leave on 10 to 15 minutes or until skin begins to redden and has a tingling sensation.
7. Encourage patient to drink plenty of liquids.
8. A warm or cool shower afterwards promotes rest.

Poultice

A warm moist mass of powdered herbs that is applied directly to the skin to:

1. Relieve inflammation.
2. Draw out poison from venomous bites and stings.
3. Relieve skin eruptions.
4. Promote proper cleansing and healing of affected area.

Using either fresh or dried herbs:

1. Grind the herbs to a powder.
2. Moisten the powdered herbs with hot water.
3. Pour the entire mixture into a cheesecloth.
4. For fresh herbs, simmer 2 ounces in 1-cup water for 2 to 3 minutes.
5. Pour the entire mixture into a cheesecloth.
6. Gently wash the area with soap and water.
7. Place a thin cloth over area. This herb mixture may also be applied directly to the skin when cool. Test on inner surface of wrist.
8. Cover with another cloth or towel to retain the heat.
9. Apply a fresh poultice when it cools.
10. Gently wash the area after removing the poultice.

Prickly-Pear Pad Poultice

The prickly pear is one of my favorite plants. It is both food and medicine. As a drawing poultice it can't be beat. First find a patch that seems right to you.

1. **Selecting the Pad**: After finding your cactus patch, look at the bottom of the plant for the youngest plumpest pad with the least stickers.
    a. Cut the pad free from the plant.
    b. Scrape the pad on a rough surface or use a rough surface rock to scrape and remove the stickers.
    c. One can also burn the stickers off.
2. **Prepare the Pad**:
    a. After the stickers are removed, cut off the outer rim of the pad.
    b. Slice through the middle like slicing through a bagel.
    c. This exposes the inner being.
    d. Scrape with a fingernail or knife to make the flesh juicer.
3. **Apply the Pad**:
    a. Place the juicy side on the affected areas.
    b. Wrap with gauze or if on the trail, use your neck scarf.
    c. The hydrophilic insides of the pad will absorb the liquid and therefore any poisons.
    d. The pad may have to be changed 3 - 4 times, so keep gathering and preparing.

Steam Inhalation

Inhalation consists of warm moist air brought to the mucous membranes of the respiratory tract. This treatment:

1. Relieves inflammation and congestion of the mucous membranes of the upper respiratory tract.
2. Relieves dry-throat tickle by moistening the air.
3. Loosens secretions and stimulates expectoration.
4. Relaxes muscles, relieves coughing.
5. Prevents excessive dryness of mucous membranes.
6. Relieves stress headaches.
7. Relieves clogged sinuses.
8. Relaxes the mind and calms the spirit.

CAUTION:

1. Pay attention. The water needs to boil and can scald if proper precautions are not taken.
2. Keep children and pets away while taking the treatment.
3. Be especially careful when giving treatment to children or restless patients.

Equipment:

1. Filtered or purified water
2. Kettle or pot
3. Glass or ceramic bowel or tall tea pot
4. Herbs or essential oils
5. Towel
6. To make a croup tent, open an umbrella, place sheet over umbrella to form a tent.

Directions:

1. Boil water until it steams.
2. Pour over herbs in container or add essential oils into boiled water.
3. Place towel over head so it forms a tent.
4. Lean toward the steam, being careful not to get too close.
5. Inhale slowly and deeply.
6. Treatment lasts 15 to 30 minutes.
7. If you or the patient start to feel overheated or uncomfortable, remove the towel or sheet.

RECIPES

Cayenne Liniment

WARNING: Don't burn your skin. Wear gloves. Do not place hands anywhere on the body while making the following cayenne recipes.

1. 1 TBSP Cayenne powder
2. 1 pint apple cider vinegar
3. Place in pan and simmer 10 minutes.
4. Place in previously sterilized bottle.

Cayenne Oil:

1. 1/2 tsp cayenne powder
2. 1 cup sunflower oil or olive oil
3. Place the above in a jar and mix well. If you set it in a warm place for two weeks, it will be a stronger remedy.

Gargles

1. **Cayenne and sea salt**: combine 1/4 tsp of each. Add 1 cup of hot water.
2. **Sage**: make a strong tea; remember, the longer it steeps, the stronger it becomes.
3. **Ginger**:
    a. 1 tsp ginger
    b. 1/2 cup hot water

c. 1/2 squeezed lemon

d. 1 tsp honey

Insect Repellants

1. **Citronella/Lavender mosquito repellent:**
    a. Add 1 to 2 ounces of citronella oil or lavender to 1 pint of sunflower oil.
    b. Make a strong tea (steep 30 minutes) of chamomile or mint, rub on exposed areas.
2. **Rosemary**: Combine these oils to 1-quart sunflower oil. You now have enough to share with friends.
    a. 1 oz. rosemary oil
    b. 1 oz. basil oil
    c. 1 oz. wormwood

Isotonic Eye Wash

Use distilled or boiled water.

1. 1 quart water: 1 tsp salt
2. 1 pint water: 1/2 tsp salt
3. 1 cup water: 1/4 tsp salt

Rehydration Drink

Fluid replacement and electrolyte balance

1. 1 qt boiled water—water that has been boiled for 10 minutes.
2. 1/2 tsp table salt

3. 1/2 tsp baking soda
4. 1 TBSP fructose or 15 TBSP white sugar or 3 TBSP honey or agave syrup

It is wise to keep a container full of Rehydration mix, ready for instant use.

Rice Water/Oatmeal Water

1. Cook any type of rice or oatmeal in twice as much water as usual.
2. Strain the mix. To the liquid add a dash of salt.

Cleaning: The Healthy And Zero Waste Way

ZERO WASTE means no toxins are used in manufacture and no toxic wastes are discarded into the environment. Spring is time to steam-clean carpets to kill mold fungi and bacteria that have built up during the winter. Add white vinegar to your water, 1 cup to a gallon of water. Read your labels. Better yet, save money and make your own GREEN Cleaners.

Basic Ingredients

1. Baking soda, without chlorine cleans and deodorizes. Softens water for more "suds."
2. Borax cleans and deodorizes, disinfectant, softens water.
3. Soap, biodegradable, nontoxic, liquid or bar. You can grate a bar to dissolve easier in hot water. Buy in bulk and store in a reused glass container.

4. Washing soda, cuts grease, removes stains.
5. White vinegar disinfects, lowers PH, bacteria can't live in an acid environment.

All Purpose Cleaners

1. Mix together 2 tbl spoons borax and 1 tsp. soap in 1 quart water, add lavender for fragrance and additional disinfectant. Use oil or make a strong tea.
2. Mix 1/2 cup white vinegar, 1/4 cup soap in 1 quart water

Scouring Powder

Add a mix of 1/14 cup coarse ground juniper leafs to baking soda or borax

Window Cleaner

1/2 tsp liquid soap, 1/4 cup vinegar, 2 cups water

Laundry Soap

Add 1/3 cup washing soda, 1/2 cup borax and lavender to water before adding clothes, hang in sunshine to disinfect.

Drain Cleaner

Drain maintenance once a week. Never pour grease, medication, or any toxic product down the drain. Pull out hair with the straightened end of a coat hanger. Pour 1/4 cup baking soda down the drain. Follow with 1/2 cup vinegar. When fizzing stops, flush with 1-gallon boiling water.

Wooden Cutting Boards

Clean once a week. rub with baking soda. Spray on full strength vinegar. Let set 5 minutes. Rinse.

Kitchen Appliances

1 tsp borax, 1/4 cup vinegar, 2 cups hot water. Spray on grease and wipe off.

Furniture Cleaner And Polish

3 parts vinegar to 3 parts lemon oil

vinegar dissolves and brings up dirt, oil enriches wood.

Oven Cleaner

Mix 1 cup of baking soda with 1/4 cup washing soda, then add enough water to make a paste. Wear house-cleaning gloves and then smear the paste on oven surfaces and leave on overnight. The next morning wipe off the mixture and grime and rinse all surfaces.

For The Garden

1. Pests that munch or suck leaves: ¼ to 1-cup vinegar, 1 1sp to ¼ cup liquid soap----if you need a stronger solution add ¼ cup cayenne or chili powder. Spray on leaves, and don't forget to spray UNDER the leaves.
2. Ants: Place white sugar around the yard or garden. They swarm at first but eventually stop coming. There is no nutrition in white sugar and there is residue from the chlorine used in bleaching to make it white. This is a new one for me, but it's worth a try!

3. Large Creepy crawlies: Pick off with tongs, Place in bucket. Relocate.
4. Planting tansy around trash areas will keep ants away. Powder tansy; add borax and sprinkle where you don't want ants.

For more comprehensive and specific information: The Encyclopedia of Natural Insect and Pest Control

TEA TIPS

Using leaves and flowers

1. 1 tsp dried leaves or 20 fresh leaves or flowers.
2. To steep, pour boiling water over herbs, cover.
3. The longer you steep, the stronger the taste.

Using roots, bark, or seeds

1. 1 tsp herb, 2 cups boiling water
2. Simmer 5 to 10 minutes; to make stronger.
3. Leave covered for 6 hours or overnight.

Tea Tips

Loose teas are preferred; some of the delicate and subtle flavors can be lost in tea bags. Herbs you pick yourself or that are picked by someone you know ensures that they have been gathered in a positive and thankful way, have not been irradiated, and have not been contaminated with pesticides and herbicides. Fresh herb tea from your garden is a special treat.

Teas need to be stored in an airtight container and in a cool dark place. Fresh herbs are chopped or used whole. Use 1 TBSP or 20 to 25 leaves or flowers. Crush seeds before brewing to bring out flavor. Roots are crushed or chopped. Avoid using stems for most plants. Mint stems add a stronger and more bitter taste. However, when using the southwest plant Cota, *Thelesperma spp.*, flowers, leaves, and upper stems are used.

Know your plant. Fresh or dried leaves or dried herbs can be added to black teas for additional flavor. Use pure water or filtered water. Note the difference when spring water is used. Herbal teas and sun teas go together.

1. Boil water until it is bubbling and rolling frantically.
    a. Rinse teapot or cup with hot water.
    b. Add the tea and cover with the boiling water.
    c. Cover while it steeps. This will prevent the aroma and medicinal properties from being carried away in the steam.
2. Steep 5 - 15 minutes. The longer it steeps the more medicinal it becomes and the stronger the taste. With some herbs, steeping longer may release bitter flavors from the chemical components in the plants, such as tannins or alkaloids.
3. When trying a new tea or herb, test for sensitivity by taking a small quantity first. If it makes you sick, try less or throw it away.
    a. When taking plants for therapeutic reasons, if it doesn't work, take a little more.
    b. If it still doesn't work, stop taking it.
    c. Too much can also hurt.
    d. Always take as directed.
    e. If you don't get better or if you get worse, call the healthcare professional who prescribed it.
    f. Above all, **Trust your judgment**.

4. Sweeteners can be used, honey, raw sugar, maple syrup, molasses, Stevia, or agave syrup. Milk can distort the real flavor. Artificial sweeteners such as aspartame are poison to the body. Avoid them.

Create your own personal teas

A tea for a rainy day, for those 100-degree days, to perk you up after a hard day at work, girl-talk teas, a special tea for that special someone in your life, to enhance natural desires, a relaxing tea—these are just a few suggestions. For every occasion there is a tea.

Grow your own plants for your special blends. Outdoor garden or window garden, they will brighten your life and become your friends. Seeds from native plants can be gathered or obtained from various seed companies or organizations specializing in native plants.

My Favorite Teas To Keep In The Kitchen

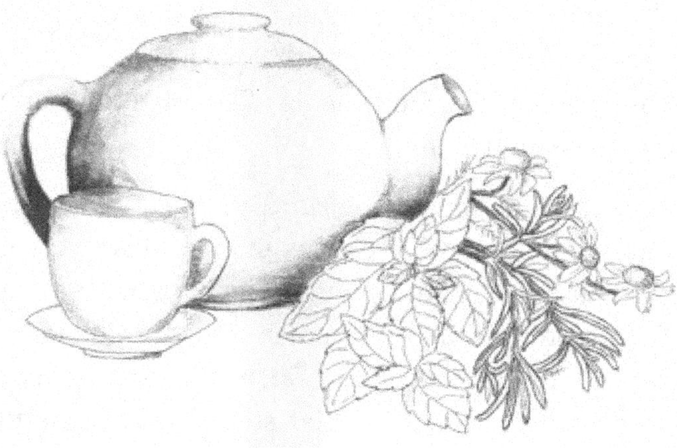

These are my favorite teas that have helped me through many unexpected circumstances. I have also included one juice that now goes with me everywhere.

1. **Black and green,** *Camellia sinensis*: Confused about these teas? All teas, both black and green, come from the same plant Camellia sinensis. The difference in the teas is the way the leaves are processed. Green tea is the least processed. Black tea is fully fermented; the leaves are exposed to air causing oxidation. This makes the leaves a rich brown color. Both are sources of Vitamin C: one cup equals 3 glasses of orange juice. Green tea is rich in fluoride and is antimicrobial, a combo that both prevents and heals gum disease. (Research has shown that gum disease can cause heart disease, stroke, and diabetes.) Both green and black teas contain tannins and flavonoids, which is why they are

helpful in skin conditions. A tried-and-true remedy for nursing mothers is placing a wet and cool tea bag on sore breasts and nipples. Tea is an ages old home treatment for burns, wounds, and sunburns. A poultice relieves itching and inflammation from insect bites. A compress stops bleeding. My Grandmother Grace used to make me a cup of tea when I had an upset stomach. Milk does not adversely affect the absorption of the constituents of tea, so add your cream and sweetener and enjoy.

2. **Catnip leaf**, *Nepeta cataria*: Every cat owner has at least one catnip mouse complete with fake whiskers lying around the house. No, I am not suggesting you raid your pet's toy. Fresh catnip from your garden is best. Although it excites cats of all ages, it is an effective muscle relaxant for us humans. Can't sleep? Mind still jogging after the day at work. Add some skullcap to the catmint, and sip on your tea while you take a nice hot lavender bath. Catnip is somewhat bitter; I add honey, stevia, or agave syrup to sweeten the taste.

3. **Chamomile flowers**, *Matricaria recutita*: When you need an herb to calm down, chamomile is the number one choice. It is effective for anxiety, palpitations, and all manifestations of stress, including insomnia. Because it has no side effects or toxicity, it is safe for babies who are suffering from colic. (Remember no honey until the child is a year old.) At first sign of cold or flu, drink Chamomile tea; it is antibacterial, especially against staph aureus and streptococcus. It also lowers fever.

4. **Chaparral**, *Larrea tridentate*: Ok. I admit few people keep Chaparral tea in their kitchen, and even fewer actually drink

it. I am never without it. Fighting an infection, drink chaparral. Do you have joint pain, arthritis? Start drinking a cup a day and notice your improvement. I find it especially useful for bronchitis and coughs. When young, my granddaughters would sleep with a glass of chaparral by their bedside. They would wake up coughing; take a drink and then sleep until morning.

5. **Ginger**, *Zingiber officinale*: Drink a cup when you have a queasy stomach or indigestion. Make a stronger cup at the first sign of cold, flu, or fever to prevent the condition from going deeper into your body. Make a strong tea of grated fresh ginger. Steep for 15 to 20 minutes, add it to a tub of hot water and take a long soak. After your bath, wrap yourself in blankets to further "sweat out" the fever. (From Brenda Morales Montoya, RN, and DOM).
6. **Lavender**, *Lavandula, officinalis*: If I had limited space, I would always have lavender and mint. Even smelling lavender energizes and lifts spirits. Stuffed up with a head cold or allergy? Inhale lavender steam. Lavender is a plant of many uses, soothes nerves, is antispasmodic and therefore useful for gas and dyspepsia, heartburn, or reflux. It is safe for infants under 6 months (I like chamomile for older children). I also keep lavender oil to use as "smelling salts." When the going gets tough, the tough sip lavender tea!
7. **Mint**, *Mentha piperita*, all mints: I am never ever without mint. My favorite is Poleo, *Mentha arvensis*, or high mountain mint. When I drink it, I am immediately transported to a high mountain stream, and I immediately relax and "cool it." The uses of this plant are many: antispasmodic, carminative, upset stomach, anti-

inflammatory, anti-bacterial. Inhale it for excessive mucus in respiratory system, calms, and quiets. In aroma therapy, it is used to increase concentration.

8. **Rosemary**, *Rosmarinus officinalis*: Can't remember what you need when you are at the grocery store? Make a list. Can't remember where have you put the list or the car keys? Time for a cup of rosemary tea. Rosemary aids the memory and helps bring the mind alert—*without* the nervous energy and unfocused actions of caffeine. It is an excellent remedy for headaches, nervousness, and nervous indigestion. No get up and go in the mornings? Forget the caffeine rush. A nice energizing rosemary bath followed by a cup of rosemary tea will energize and focus you for the day's activities. It has been used to increase poor circulation and strengthen fragile blood vessels. Oh, and don't "forget" its use as a hair tonic.
9. **Rosehip,** *Rosa spp.*: Nothing is more beautiful than the wild rose. It can be found in all altitudes, but most frequently in mountainous areas, streamside, and moist meadows. The flowers mature into hips, those little fruits that turn from green- yellow to a translucent dark red. Rosehips are a local and inexpensive source of Vitamin C. They have 60-times the Vitamin C as citrus fruit. They are also a source of bioflavonoid that aids in the absorption of Vitamin C and iron. The seeds can be ground into meal and added to cereals and muffins. They are a source of Vitamin E, sulfur, and unsaturated fats. Add a little cinnamon and enjoy on a cold winter day.

I prefer to prevent or heal *dis*-ease using natural remedies because there are fewer side effects, and I save money.

SPICES

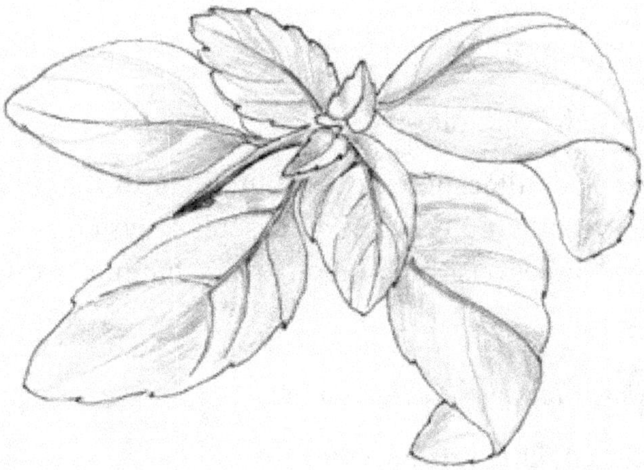

Tumeric, Curcuma longa

Aloe Vera, *Aloe barbadensis*

Part used: Leaf

Use: Heals cuts and burns. The juice soothes and heals an irritated digestive tract. Laxative use of aloe is not recommended. antibacterial

Anise, *Pimpinella anisum*

Part used: Seeds

Use: Aids digestion, colic, gas, carminative, coughs, promotes expectoration, bronchitis, spasmodic asthma, the oil is used as antiseptic, repels insects

Basil, *Ocimum basilicum*

Part used: Leaf

Uses: Carminative, mild nervous disorders, fresh leaves placed on stings draws poison out, insect repellant, mild antiseptic

Bay, *Laurus nobilis*

Part used: Leaf, oil

Uses: Aids digestion, colic, diuretic, arthritis, inflammations, antioxidant, protects cardiovascular system, bacterial and fungal infections, high blood sugar, inhibits growth of cancer cells

Cardamon, *Elettaria cardamomum*

Part used: Dried ripe seeds

Uses: Digestive system: carminative, dyspepsia, indigestion, helps stop belching, vomiting, respiratory system: added to milk to neutralize the mucus forming properties, expectorant circulatory, calms nervous system, detoxes caffeine, calms nervous stomach

Cayenne, *Capsicum annum (Chili)*

Part used: Whole fruit

Uses: Anti-viral, helpful in congestive heart failure, counter irritant, diaphoretic, increases circulation by moving blood from center of body to periphery, aids blood flow to mucosa, stimulates production of hydrochloric acid in the stomach, increases salivary and intestinal juices, doesn't irritate lower digestive tract, reduces uric acid, diuretic, relieves pain.

Celery Seed, *Apium graveolens*

Part used: Seed, herb and root

Uses: Carminative, diuretic, stomach tonic, calms nerves, good for hysteria, promotes sleep

Chives, *Allium schoenoprasum*

Part used: Leaf

Uses: Stimulates appetite, digestive aid, mildly antibiotic, reduces blood pressure, tones the stomach

high concentrations of Vitamins A and C, high in iron and sulfur, calcium, magnesium, potassium, thiamine, and niacin

Chocolate, *Theobroma cacao*

Part Used: Bean, bark, made into butter/fat

Uses: Mild stimulant to nervous system, asthma, bronchitis, respiratory distress, anemia antioxidant, calms moods, and for those intimate moments, increases virility

Cilandro, *Coriandrum sativum*

Part used: Fruit and leaf

Use: Stimulant, aromatic, carminative, anesthetizes stomach, digestive aid, soothing laxative, soothes cramping, seeds as sedative

Cinnamon, *Cinnamomum zeylanicum*

Part used: Dried bark

Use: High in calcium, menstrual cramps, digestive aid, flatulence, diabetes, astringent, diarrhea, antibacterial, inhibits e-coli, staph aureus, and candida albicans

Citrus, *Citrus aurantium, citrus vulgaris (lemon, lime, orange, etc)*

Part used: Fruit, peel, and flowers

Uses: Flowers, anxiety and nervous depression, stimulates digestive juices, diuretic, fruit high in Vitamin C, antioxidant

Cilantro, *Eugenia aromatica*

Part used: Underdeveloped flowers

Use: Anesthetic, germicide, antiseptic, anthelmintic

Coffee, *Coffea Arabica*

Part used: Berries, seeds, and caffeine

Use: Stimulates the central nervous system, has a "wake up' effect on the brain, diuretic

Cumin, *Cuminum* cyminum

Part used: Seeds

Use: Curry and spice mixtures, carminative, and antispasmodic

Dill, *Anethum graveolens*

Part used: Leaf, seeds

Use: Aromatic, carminative, stomach tonic, colic, sour gassy stomach

Epazote, *Chenopodium ambrosioides*

Part used: Leaf

Use: Classic seasoning for beans, prevents gas, stimulates milk for nursing mothers, menstrual stimulant, anthelmintic

Fennel, *Foeniculum vulgare*

Part used: Seeds, leaf

Use: Stimulant diaphoretic, loosens bronchial secretions, emmenagogue, increases secretion of milk, in India used to keep insects away, antispasmodic

Fenugreek, *Trigonella foenum-graecum*

Part used: Seeds

Use: Diabetes, inflammations of the stomach and intestines, prevent fevers, poultices for abscesses, boils, carbuncles, contains female estrogen, folk remedy for breast enlargement

Garlic, *Allium sativum*

Part used: Bulb

Use: Diaphoretic, diuretic, expectorant, antibiotic, lung disorders, promotes digestion, helps balance blood sugar, expels worms, germicidal, moves blood stagnation and clots, opens vessels, balances blood pressure, protects against the heavy metals cadmium and mercury, antioxidant, helps prevent chromosome breakage, increases bile secretion, builds cells, calms nerves, immune stimulant, normalizes calcium metabolism, antibiotic especially gram-negative bacteria, protects against vampires

Ginger, *Zingiber officinale*

Part used: Root, fresh is best, at least a year old

Uses: Stimulant, carminative, dyspepsia, gas, colic, cramps, nausea, diaphoretic, rubefacient

***CAUTION**: do not use if person has gastric ulcers*

Lavender, *Lavandula officinalis*

Part used: Dried flowers

Uses: Burns, stings, headache, coughs, colds, strong antibacterial action, kills streptococcus, chest infections, sedative, calms anxiety and tension, spasms of digestive tract, nervous headaches, in massage oil relaxes muscles

Marjoram, *Origanum majorana*

Part used: Leaves

Uses: Asthma, indigestion, arthritis, toothache, antioxidant, antifungal

Mustard, *Brassica alba*

Part used: Seeds

Uses: Counterirritant, bronchitis, sore throat, stimulant, diuretic, emetic

Nutmeg, *Myristica fragrans*

Part used: dried kernel of the seed

Uses: Tonic, to flavor medicines, flatulence, nausea and vomiting

Oregano, *Origanum vulgare*

Part used: Leaf

Uses: Indigestion, tonic, coughs, headache, promotes menses, poultice to soothe painful swollen joints, antiseptic

Oregano De La Sierra, *Monarda didyma*

Part used: Flowers, leaves

Uses: Leaves in cooking, flowers garnish salads, coughs, sore throats, nausea, flatulence, and menstrual cramps

Parsley, *Carum petroselinum*

Part used: Root, seed, leaves

Uses: Diuretic, poultice of leaves for bites and stings, high in calcium and Vitamins A and C, arthritis, antispasmodic

Peppercorns, *Piper nigrum*

Part used: Seeds

Uses: Stimulates taste buds, promotes gastric secretions, are ground and mixed with honey each morning for excess mucus and sore throats

Peppermint (any of the mints), *Mentha piperita*

Part used: Leaves and flowers

Uses: Antispasmodic, nausea, flatulence, diaphoretic, heartburn, antiseptic, anesthetic, disinfectant, neuralgic headaches, palpitations of heart, hysteria, stimulates circulation, inhale oil for chest complaints, disliked by rats

Rosemary, *Rosmarinus officinalis*

Part used: Herb, root

Uses: Tonic, astringent, diaphoretic, stimulant, prevention of baldness (nutrition and external), dandruff, depression, headaches, stimulates brain and nervous system, improves memory

Sage, *Salvia officinalis*

Part used: Leaves, whole herb

Uses: Stimulant, astringent, tonic and carminative, stimulates menses, relieves nervous headache, removes mucus from respiratory tract

Savory, *Satureja hortensis*

Part used: Herb

Uses: Culinary, carminative, colic, and gas, First Aid for wasp and bee stings

Taragon, *Artemisia drancunculus*

Part used: Herb, root

Uses: Tonic, induces appetite, root used for toothache

Tea, *Camellia sinensis, black or green*

Part used: Leaves

Uses: Green tea is least processed, both black and green are sources of Vitamin C, antimicrobial, anti-inflammatory, astringent, burns, sunburns, gum disease, antioxidant, prevents dental carries, improves beneficial intestinal flora, contains caffeine (30mg to 90mg per cup) for alertness

Thyme, *Thymus vulgaris*

Part used: Herb

Uses: Anthelmintic, antispasmodic, diaphoretic, expectorant, sedative, bronchitis, and laryngitis; oil of thyme contains thymol used in bath as stimulate of circulation, relieves nervous exhaustion, is antiseptic

Tumeric, *Curcuma longa*

Part used: Dried rhizome

Uses: Stimulates flow of bile from liver, stomach disorders, liver ailments, jaundice, increases circulation, antibiotic, anti-inflammatory, improves intestinal flora, blood purifier, promotes proper metabolism in body, tonic to skin; powder burned to keep away mosquitoes

My Favorite First Aid Plants

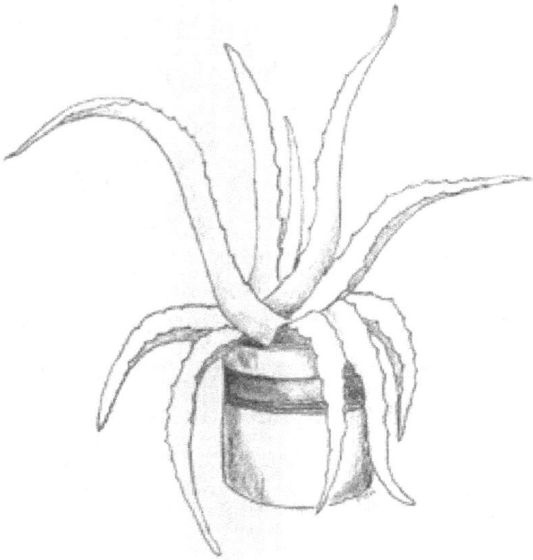

Aloe vera

These are my favorite First Aid plants. Very hard to choose. But aloe vera and chaparral are already in my kitchen, ready for use if needed. Choose the top 10 plants you might need for First Aid and minor ailments. Whatever they are, keep them as teas, tinctures, or salves, have an organic supply and be ready for anything.

1. **Aloe Vera**, *Aloe barbadensis*: Technically, this is not a tea. However, I drink its juice daily, and always have a plant available for burns. The gel heals cuts and burns and the juice soothes and heals an irritated digestive tract. It is anti-bacterial and anti-inflammatory. This plant has many nutritional compounds in abundance. It is high in magnesium, the main compound in many of the over-the-counter heartburn medicines.

2. **Aspen,** *Populus tremuloides*, or **Cottonwood**, *Populus spp.:* Aspen likes the high mountains, way above its desert cousin, the Cottonwood. Both contain populin that converts to salicin. Both are anti-inflammatory, reduce fever, relieve pain. Neither one triggers an allergy response or causes stomach bleeding. In the Spring gather the buds, they are the strongest medicine. In the summer the leaves can be used. Autumn to late Fall, gather bark. Can be used as tea, tincture or salve. Do not take internally if you are taking anticoagulants, like coumadin or low dose aspirin.

3. **Calendula**, *Calendula officinalis*: A lovely garden plant from the Mediterranean area. She is easy to grow from seeds, liking rich composted soil and mulch. Since ancient times Her flowers and petals have been used to heal wounds. Calendula is bactericide, antiseptic and has anti-inflammatory properties. Soak a compress in a strong flower tea and use with wounds to prevent infections and aid wound healing. The salve soothes the cut, scrapes and abrasions of the little ones and soon the tears stop.

4. **Chili,** *Capsicum annum*: Food and medicine, the plant that has gone around the world, delighting taste buds, and maintaining health everywhere it goes. It is packed with power, likes free radicals, and scavenges them, aids digestion, high in vitamins, especially A and C, moves blood from center of the body and takes the load off the heart, increases circulation to the hands and feet, can block pain for up to 8 hours. Salsa and blue corn chips! Yummy!

5. **Comfrey,** *Symphytum officinale***:** She is centuries old but looks strong and healthy in my garden. Down through the

ages and varying civilizations she has healed wounds and promoted new cell and tissue growth, including bones and ligaments. A poultice of the leaves or tea from the leaves can help arthritic joints and treat skin conditions like eczema. The root is also used, but then it destroys the whole plant. Both leaves and roots contain Allantoin one of the main healing chemicals in this plant.

6. **Dandelion,** *Taraxacum officinale*: What a wonderous plant, beauty, first food for early bees, food for humans and medicine. So why do people spend millions of dollars trying to exterminate them? What they are doing is putting poison into their own soil and water. Besides that, the dandelion is an ACCURATE weather forecaster, folding up its petals if rain threatens. All parts are edible, flowers, leaves, roots. Roots contain iron and help build up red blood. They are diuretic, but don't deplete the body of potassium. The leaves are nutritious and can also be used as a drawing poultice.

7. **Echinacea,** *Echinacea angustifolia*: A favorite first aid plant from the Plains of East and Central US. It is active against bacteria, viruses, and yeasts, stimulates growth of new tissue, stimulates the immune system, neutralizes the bite of the Brown Recuse spider and other poisonous critters. It has no toxic side effects and there are only very rare allergic reactions. Take this when you first start feeling sick. It is not for long term use and if used in large quantities for a long time it can cause depression.

8. **Mullein,** *Verbascum thapsus*: Another naturalized Earth citizen. It was brought in seed form from Europe. Today it can be found in the garden, mountains, and roadways. The flowers are anti-viral and are effective against herpes

simplex. The leaves have long been a remedy for the lungs as demulcent, expectorant and astringent. The leaves are found in most herbal tobaccos. Inhaling the smoke helps to relieve asthma. The boiled leaves are used as a poultice for painful joints. When out in nature and nature calls, the soft fuzzy leaves are useful.

9. **Osha,** *Lingusticum porterii*: I learned about Osha when I emigrated to New Mexico and now I always have some, at home and in my travel first aid kit. It is sacred to the Native People of the Southwest. When I wildcraft it, I pray, give thanks, offer tobacco, and ask permission to take a few roots home to use as medicine. It is an antibiotic and immune strengthening and is very useful for lung conditions and coughs. As a salve it prevents infections and aids healing. It is used for arthritis, sore muscles and misc. aches and pains. Use it for a gargle for sore throats. Carrying a piece with you when hiking keeps snakes away.

10. **Plantain,** *Plantago major, lanceolata*: Plantago major, lanceolate: Another useful naturalized citizen who came to America with the early pioneers. So glad that happened! Walking along and you get stung by a bee. Look around you and you will soon spot one of the plantains. Pick a leaf, chew it and place it on the bite site. It will draw out the venom and soothe the area. This plant stops both internal and external bleeding. A compress of the tea soothes irritated inflamed skin and membranes. The seeds are used to stop diarrhea. Diarrhea on the trail isn't pleasant, in fact it isn't pleasant anywhere.

11. **Rose,** *Rosa spp*: Every part of the lovely rose can be used for food and medicine. Traditionally New Mexicans used the

flower petals as a wash to relieve tired inflamed eyes. The rose is astringent and can be used for diarrhea. Gargle with a strong tea to relieve a sore throat. Rosehip tea contains Vit. C, antioxidants and can strengthen blood vessels and support the adrenal glands. And you thought she was just "Vase candy."

12. **Yarrow,** *Achillea millefolium*: Mountain meadows abound with this lovely flower. It is found throughout the West. Collect and use the whole flowering plant including the rootlet. So, many uses. It is a trail remedy to stop bleeding on cuts and abrasion. Drink the tea as stomach tonic that aids digestion. Made strong enough it will stimulate sweating and bring down a fever.

HERBAL INSECT REPELLANTS

DEET: N, N-DIDDDETHYL-META-TOLUAMIDE

This popular insect repellant was developed in 1046 by the US Army to protect soldiers in the field, forest, and jungle. It became available for public use in 1957. Deet blocks the insects' olfactory receptors. They can't find you by scent. However, it is also a neuro toxin, a chemical that adversely affects the nervous system for both insects and mammals, including humans. When it is mixed with a sunscreen product it causes more to be absorbed into the body. If you drink alcohol and apply sunscreen that contains Deet you absorb twice as much. Symptoms of exposure:

1. Irritated, painful watery eyes.
2. Irritated red rash on skin.
3. Some people experience seizures.

We do not know the effects of chronic long-term exposure, like applying small amounts on the skin daily. It should never be applied to the skin of infants and small children. There are now many commercial natural products to repel insects, or you can make your own, choosing from this list of common herbs and plants that are effective and can be used safely indoors and outside.

A star indicates for external use only and to use only outdoors.

- Basil
- Bay leaves
- Camphor weed
- Catnip

- Cayenne pepper
- Cedar
- Chamomile
- Citronella, found in a variety of plants
- Cloves
- Cypress
- Eucalyptus leaves
- Feverfew
- Garlic
- Lavender
- Orange
- Patchouli oil
- *Pennyroyal
- *Pyrethrum, will kill beneficial as well as the pests
- Rosemary
- Sage
- Sassafras
- Tansy
- *Tobacco, cultivated, wild or organic commercial
- Turmeric, burned as a powder in India to repel insects.
- Wormwood

BASIC FIRST AID KITS

Basic First Aid kits for home, car, camping, and hiking can be purchased or assembled by the individual or family. A First Aid book is essential. When selecting or making kits, keep this in mind:

1. Kit is large enough to meet your needs.
2. Arrange contents so items can be found quickly; have a list of those contents.
3. Keep all medicine out of reach of children.
4. Excessive sun / heat will deteriorate both pharmaceuticals and botanicals.
5. Check the contents every 2 to 3 months for outdated or damaged supplies.

Basic Supplies For Kit

1. First Aid book
2. Band-aids, assorted sizes
3. Non-stick dressings, assorted sizes
4. Butterfly bandages or Steri-Strips, assorted sizes
5. Gauze pads, 2x2, 4x4
6. Sterile eye patches
7. Roller gauze, 2 inches and 4 inches
8. Elastic wrap (Ace Bandages) 2 inches and 4 inches
9. Triangular bandages

10. Adhesive tape
11. Bandage compresses (ABD pads)
12. Cotton swabs
13. Cotton balls
14. Safety pins
15. Steel sewing needles
16. Paper clips
17. Scissors
18. Tweezers
19. Soap
20. Matches, waterproof or in watertight container
21. Snakebite kit, with instructions in print you can read.
22. Thermometer, a temporal scanner is preferred.
23. Alcohol, hydrogen peroxide
24. Masks
25. Gloves
26. Baggies to hold blood and infectious waste.

Other Helpful Additions To First Aid Kit

1. Syrup of Ipecac: A botanical extract from the *Cephaelis Ipecacuanha* plant of South America. It is a natural irritant to the stomach that safely induces vomiting in 20 minutes.
2. RESCUE REMEDY: Bach flower remedy for cases of shock, panic, and stress.

3. Arnica: homeopathic pills, salve, or as liniment to reduce swelling from injuries.
4. First Aid salves, soothing and antibiotic.
5. Clay, green or gray to draw out poisons from bite or sting.
6. Pain reliever, what you and your family usually takes.
7. Resuscitator mask, oral airway

KITCHEN EQUIPMENT

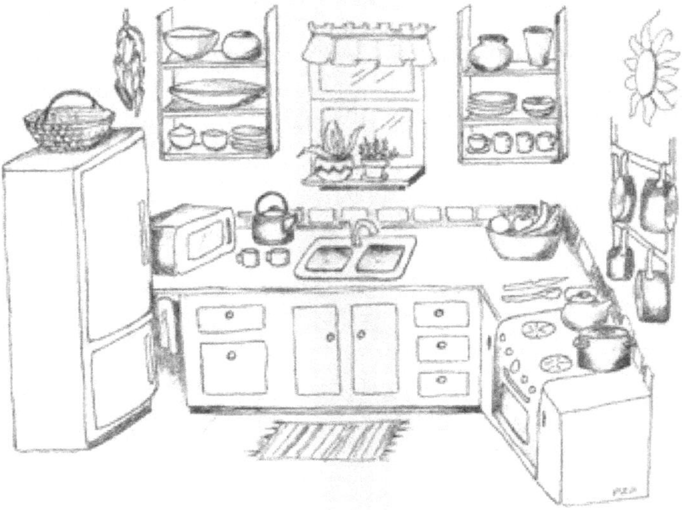

Do not use aluminum. Constituents from some plants can react to form aluminum compounds. Aluminum can leech into the liquids of foods being cooked. Foods cooked in aluminum produce a chloride poison that neutralizes the digestive juices, making them less acidic, and therefore reduces digestion in the stomach. Excess aluminum is deposited in the brain and nervous system. It will continue to accumulate there. Accumulation of aluminum salts in the brain has been implicated in seizures and reduced mental faculties. Autopsies have found that the brains of Alzheimer's victims have four times the normal amounts of aluminum. The aging brain is less able to process aluminum. In 2020, a study published in the *Journal of Alzheimer's Disease* links human exposure to aluminum with Alzheimer's disease. The controversy continues. Why take chances?

Basic Kitchen Equipment

Some of these may be useful in emergency situations.

1. Aloe Vera plant
2. Wooden spoons
3. Spatula
4. Sharp knives
5. Knife sharpener: Nothing can cause more problems than a dull knife.
6. Cutting boards: Clean well after using. Pour vinegar on the board; let it set for about 15 minutes; rinse to help kill and remove bacteria.
7. Garlic press, (great tool to get all the juices)
8. Grater
9. Spice and seed grinder
10. Kitchen thermometer
11. Strainers
12. Tea balls
13. Vegetable scrub brush
14. Wire whisk
15. Juicer: This is major investment; therefore, research, talk with people who use them before making your decision.
16. Hot pads
17. Heat absorbent pads
18. Apron with pockets

OTHER KITCHEN NECESSITIES

Apple Cider Vinegar

Apple cider vinegar (ACV) is made by crushing fresh organic apples and allowing them to ferment in wooden barrels. When ACV is mature, it contains a dark, cloudy foam called "Mother." Vinegars that contain "Mother" have enzymes and minerals that other vinegars have lost due to over processing and overheating. ACV contains these minerals and trace elements: potassium, calcium, magnesium, phosphorous, chlorine, sodium, sulfur, copper, iron, silicon, and fluorine; these are all vital for a healthy balanced body. My father drank apple cider vinegar, honey, and water daily upon rising. He was a healthy man who rarely had a cold.

Apple cider vinegar contains 55% acetic acid, which makes it a mild acid with a pH of 2 - 3. (ph. is a measure of acidity, with 1 being the most acidic and 7 being neutral) Its disinfectant properties have been verified by numerous scientific studies.

These are a few of the circumstances that benefit from taking ACV:

1. Reduce sinus infections and sore throats.
2. Cure skin conditions such as acne.
3. Strengthen the immune system.
4. Improve digestion.
5. Increase metabolism.
6. Prevent kidney stones and urinary tract infections.
7. Help lower cholesterol.

8. Help balance blood sugar.

As with everything, there are precautions:

1. I do not recommend taking vinegar tablets or capsules; these are very concentrated, and if lodged in throat or esophagus can cause tissue damage.
2. Always dilute any acid drink, taking them "straight" on a long-term basis can erode teeth enamel, giving teeth a yellowish look and making them more sensitive to heat and cold.
3. Moderation: The key to taking any vitamin or mineral supplement, food, or herbal product is moderation or as directed.
4. If you are allergic to apples—don't take apple cider vinegar.

I always have one day of the week when I take NO vitamins or supplements, giving the liver a break. One of the many jobs of the liver is breaking down everything that comes into our body into a usable or excretable form. I may take ACV for several months then switch to water and chlorophyll or only drink aloe vera juice for a few months.

Baking Soda

Sodium bicarbonate or sodium hydrogen carbonate is a chemical compound with the formula NaHCO2. It is a white crystalline powder that has a slight alkaline taste. The natural mineral form is known as nahcolite. It is also produced artificially. One of its values is its acid-neutralizing properties. It is used in cooking where it reacts with other components to release carbon dioxide as in helping dough to rise. A paste of baking soda and water can be an effective cleaning and scrubbing agent. Keep it in the kitchen to use it to smother a small fire. Its medicinal uses include acting as an antacid to treat acid indigestion and heartburn. It can treat cases of acidosis, and taken in a warm bath, it can reduce itching. A paste placed on an insect sting will draw the poison out.

Honey

PRECAUTION: Not for children under one year. Their underdeveloped digestive systems cannot handle the natural presence of botulism endospores.

Honey is a mixture of monosaccharide sugars and other compounds, such as digestive enzymes and compounds thought to function as antioxidants. Honey contains trace amounts of B Vitamins, folate, Vitamin C, and the minerals calcium, iron, magnesium, phosphorus, potassium, sodium, and zinc. Each batch of honey is different, depending on the flowers the bees visit. Things to know when buying, storing, and using honey:

1. Fresh honey flows from a knife in a straight flow.
2. If honey is transparent, it has likely been heated and has lost its value.
3. Types
    a. Best if certified ORGANIC.
    b. Comb honey: Honey still in the original comb.
    c. Raw honey: Extracted in temperatures under 120°F. May contain some pollen and pieces of wax.
    d. Strained: Honey passed thru a mesh material to remove particles.

4. Storage:
    a. Store in the dark. Direct sunlight can destroy enzymes.
    b. Store in a dry area. Honey can absorb moisture and might start fermenting.
    c. Three years is the max it can be stored.
    d. Use glass or ceramic containers to avoid absorption of heavy metals.
    e. Heating up to 98.6 °F causes it to lose its nutritive value and antimicrobial qualities.
    f. Do not microwave honey; it reduces enzyme activity and nutritive content—*however,* microwaving does increase shelf life.

Honey has been shown to be a cough suppressant, immune-system booster, and free-radical cleanser. Research indicates that it promotes blood sugar control and heightens insulin sensitivity. With its low water content, acidic properties (PH 3.2 – 4.5), and its dilute hydrogen peroxide content, it kills infection-causing organisms. It is especially effective against staphylococcus aurous, an infection that can mutate into methylin-resistant staphylococcus aurous (MRSA), which is now spread in both hospitals and communities and can be deadly.

Olive Oil

The seeds of the olive tree, *Olea europaea*, are pressed to make olive oil. Olive oil is a source of Vitamin E, trace elements, and unsaturated fats. It is nourishing as well as being a demulcent, lubricant, and laxative. It is calming, moistening, and promotes both digestion and the healing of wounds. Extra virgin oil is the least processed.

Salt

Sodium and chloride ions are the two major components of salt. Salt is essential for all human and animal life. When our ancient ancestors left the sea to live on land, they took some of the sea with them enclosed in their bodies. We are actually an inland sea. Salt flavor is one of our basic tastes.

Salt plays an intricate role in regulating the water content of our bodies. Too much or too little can tip the scale and create an imbalance that can lead to death. A deficiency produces muscle cramps, dizziness, and fatal neurological problems.

Excessive intake has been linked to asthma, edema, heartburn, osteoporosis, duodenal ulcers, gastric ulcers, gastric cancer, high blood pressure, cardiac enlargement, and cardiovascular disease.

Forms of salt

1. Unrefined sea salt: Contains trace minerals, but little iodine. Tastes slightly bitter.
2. Refined salt: The refining process removes most other minerals.
3. Table salt: 99% sodium chloride and 1% anti-caking agents, to make it free flowing. Often sodium aluminosilicate and aluminum-calcium silicate are used—check your labels carefully.
4. Iodized salt: Helps reduce the chance of iodine deficiency.

5. Sea salt: If using sea salt, you must add kelp powder to the salt, include kelp in your diet, or take kelp supplements. Most commercial sea salt comes with iodine added.

Sunflower Oil

The sunflower, *Helianthus annuus*, is a native of Mexico and Peru. Sunflower seeds are a great source of essential fatty acids necessary to produce prostaglandins, the hormone-like compounds that regulate every function in the body at the molecular level. It is high in linoleic and oleic acids and is a combination of mono-unsaturated and polyunsaturated fats with a low saturated fat level. It is high in Vitamin E, lecithin, and carotenoids. There are many healthful reasons to use sunflower oil. It has been shown to have cholesterol-reducing properties. Vitamin E is an antioxidant that protects the heart. Research has shown that linoleic and oleic acids are beneficial in diabetes. Sunflower oil helps the skin retain moisture while providing a protective barrier that resists infection. It is very soothing to the skin. The seeds are diuretic and have expectorant properties. It has been used in the treatment of bronchial, laryngeal, and pulmonary conditions, colds, and coughs. It is my favorite, and my kitchen always has a ready supply.

Washing Soda

Washing soda is a chemical compound that contains sodium carbonate. It can be used to remove stubborn stains like blood, tea, and coffee, as well as greasy buildup on pans. The washing soda binds to the minerals that make water hard, thus removing dirt by allowing the detergent to be absorbed into the fibers of material. It is often used in products that are used to treat "hard water." It is

NOT baking soda, although they are related. It is NOT for internal use.

Water

Everything originated in water. Everything will be sustained by water.

- Johann Wolfgang Goethe, German philosopher, and poet

Water sustains all life on Earth, and Earth is the only planet in our solar system known to have liquid water on its surface. Two thirds or 70% of our body's total weight is water. Our body is designed to run on water. We function more efficiently when we are properly hydrated. Eight, 8-ounce glasses of water are the minimal amount to drink per day. This varies with activity, climate, and season. Proper hydration can prevent headaches, keep blood pressure from going dangerously low (blood pressure varies with blood volume), aids digestion, and helps kidneys regulate body fluid balance. Too much water loss decreases blood flow to the brain and causes headache, nausea, confusion, and eventual collapse. Even mild dehydration slows down metabolism as much as 3%. Lack of water is the number one cause of daytime fatigue. Want to lose weight? Drink water. Having trouble focusing on the computer screen or reading a printed page? Can't do basic math? Memory a bit fuzzy? How much water did you drink today? Even a 2% drop in body water can cause these symptoms.

So, relax, sit in your favorite chair, and enjoy a nice, cool, refreshing glass of pure, uncontaminated water.

Measuring Dry Herbs

The best way to measure ounces is with a simple pan-balance scale. These can be purchased from scientific supply stores and some drugstores. Kitchen scales are available for under twenty dollars.

U.S. And Metric Measures

1/2 teaspoon	=	30 drops				
1 teaspoon	=	60 drops	=	5 milliliters		
3 teaspoons	=	1 tablespoon	=	1/2 fluid ounce		
2 tablespoons	=			1 fl. ounce		
4 tablespoons	=	1/4 cup	=	2 fl. ounces		
8 tablespoons	=	1/2 cup	=	4 fl. ounces		
16 tablespoons	=	1 cup	=	8 fl. ounces		
2 cups	=	1 pint	=	16 fl. Ounces	=	1/2 liter
4 cups	=	1 quart	=	2 pints	=	1 liter
4 quarts	=	1 gallon	=	3.7 liters		
16 ounces dry	=	1 pound				

GLOSSARY

ANALGESIC: Relieves pain

ANESTHETIC: Agent that causes temporary and reversible loss of sensation

ANTHELMINTIC: Kills worms

ANTIBIOTIC (antibacterial): Inhibits growth of bacteria or kills on contact.

ANTICOAGULANT: A substance that stops blood from clotting

ANTI-INFLAMMATORY: An agent, herb, drug or food that reduces signs of inflammation such as swelling, tenderness, fever, pain

ANTIOXIDANT: Prevents oxidation or rancidity: A preservative. Antioxidants protect our cells from the effects of free radicals. Free radicals are molecules produced from the breakdown of environmental exposures like tobacco, cleaning chemicals, substances used in chemotherapy for cancer, pesticides, and radiation. Free radicals can damage cells and researchers think they play a role in heart disease, cancer, and other diseases.

ANTISEPTIC: Prevents or retards growth of bacteria

ANTISPASMODIC: Relieves or prevents spasms, usually of the smooth muscle of the intestinal tract or uterus

ANTIVIRAL: An agent that kills a virus or suppresses its ability to replicate and produce toxins

ASTRINGENT: Causes constriction of tissues and is used to stop bleeding, secretions, etc.

BITTER: Releases digestive hormones that stimulate the appetite and flow of digestive juices

BPA, Bisphenol A: an organic compound used to make polycarbonate plastic and epoxy resins. It is known to be estrogenic. There are concerns regarding exposure of fetuses, infants, and young children. In September 2010 Canada became the first country to declare BPA a toxic substance. It is banned in baby bottles.

BRONCHIAL DILATOR: Something that opens the bronchial passages and allows more oxygen to enter.

CARBUNCLE: A severe abscess or multiple boils in the kin. Typically infected with staphylococcus bacteria.

CARMINATIVE: Relieves and removes gas from intestinal tract

CHOP: Quick heavy strokes using a knife or other sharp tool to cut food into irregular bite-sized pieces.

COAGULATION: In the body it is the process in which a blood clot is formed. Without this process we could bleed to death. Too much clotting can occlude blood vessels causing strokes or heart attacks. Balance is the key.

COLIC: Severe stomach cramps

COMPRESS: External application of herbs that is used to treat superficial ailments, stimulate circulation of blood or lymph, relieve colic, muscle spasms, reduce inflammation, reduce fevers

CONTRACTURE: A condition of shortening and hardening of muscles, tendons or other tissues often leading to deformity and rigidity of joints

COUNTERIRRITANT/RUBAFACIENT: Induces superficial irritation to relieve another irritation or to stimulate circulation.

CROUP: A respiratory, upper airway condition triggered by an acute virus infection. The trachea or the vocal cords swell causing a barky cough. It is usually found in children 6 months to 3 years old. A cool mist humidifier, steam treatment or croup tent are helpful. A croup tent concentrates humidity which helps prevent the loss of water from the child's body causing dehydration and thins the phlegm making it easier to expel, therefore clearing the lung airways making it easier to breathe.

DEMULCENT: Soothes and softens

DECOCTION: A tea that is boiled slowly for 15 to 20 minutes, usually of roots, bark, or large seeds

DIALYSIS: Mechanical purification of blood as a substitute for the normal function of the kidney

DIAPHORETIC: Promotes sweating

DICE: To cut food into small uniform pieces (cubes)

DIURETIC: Increases flow of urine

DOUBLE BOILER: A way of cooking without direct heat. A bottom saucepan is filled with water and the top pan with the mixture to be cooked.

DYSPEPSIA: Upset stomach, heartburn

EDEMA: Swelling caused by too much fluid trapped in the body's tissues. It is most often seen in the legs and feet.

EMETIC: Promotes vomiting

EMMENAGOGUE: Stimulates menstrual flow.

EMOLLIENT: Soothes and softens

EXPECTORANT: Stimulates the removal of mucus from lungs

FERMENTATION: The conversion of sugars into alcohols or acids using yeast, bacteria, or both. This process is used for making certain beverages such as: cider, mead, beer, and wine, and to preserve foods: sauerkraut, kimchi, yogurt, or vinegar.

FLATULENCE: Expelled gas from the colon

GANGRENE: Localized death and decomposition of body tissue, resulting from either obstructed circulation or bacterial infection.

GARGLE: The process in which one bubbles a liquid in the mouth as the head tilts backward, goes to the upper part of the throat. It is used for: cleaning the throat, soothing irritated and inflamed mucus membranes, and removing bacteria and viruses from the throat.

GMO: Genetically modified organisms

GRATE: To cut into very small pieces using a grater

HAEMOSTATIC: Stops internal or external bleeding

INFECTION: The colonization of a host organism by a pathogen. The infecting organism interferes with the normal functioning of the host, can lead to death.

INFLAMMATION: The body's natural response to infections, damaged cells, or irritants. The body tries to remove the injurious stimuli and to initiate the healing process. Inflammation is not the same as infection.

INFUSION: A method of brewing tea, in which boiling water is poured over a plant, leaves, or flowers.

KETOACIDOSIS: A complication of diabetes that occurs when the body cannot use sugar as a fuel and fat is used instead. The by-products of fat breakdown are called ketones and build up in the body. Ketones are poisonous. Warning signs: deep rapid breathing, dry skin, and mouth, flushed face, fruity breath, nausea and vomiting, stomach pain. The treatment is to correct the high blood sugar levels. Untreated ketoacidosis can lead to severe illness or death.

LAXATIVE: Relieves constipation

LINIMENT: A medicated liquid that is rubbed on the skin, usually to relieve pain, muscle aches, and arthritis.

MASH: To crush, beat or squeeze a food into a soft state

NERVINE: Stops nervousness and irritability

NETI POT: A device used for irrigating the nasal passages. It can be made of ceramic, glass, metal, or plastic. Typically, it has a spout attached near the bottom, often with a handle on the opposite side.

OINTMENT/SALVE: Semi-solid preparations made from beeswax and oil and organic herbal material that are applied to the skin.

PALPITATIONS: Abnormality of heartbeat that causes awareness of its beating

POULTICE: A warm moist mass of powdered herbs that is applied directly to the skin to: relieve inflammation, draw out poison from venomous bites and stings, skin eruptions, promote proper cleansing and healing of affected area.

PUREE: To puree is to make a smooth creamy substance of liquidized or crushed fruit or vegetables

RUBAFACIENT: A counterirritant: induces superficial irritation to relieve another irritation; stimulates circulation to an area.

SEDATIVE: Sleep inductive

SIMMER: To cook a liquid at just below the boiling point

STEAM INHALATION: Inhalation of warm moist air into the mucus membranes of the respiratory tract.

STEEP: Soak in water or other liquid to extract flavor or to soften an object, such as plant leaf. To soak or saturate (cloth) in water or other liquid.

STERILIZE: Make something free from bacteria or other living microorganisms

STRAIN: To separate liquids from solids by passing through a sieve or cheesecloth

TINCTURE: Water and alcohol concentration of a plant, an extract.

URIC ACID: An almost insoluble compound, which is a breakdown product of nitrogenous metabolism.

RESOURCES

American Academy of Orthopedic Surgeons, www.aaos.org

Auerbach, Paul, MD, Medicine for The Outdoors, 1986

Bigfoot, Peter; Zella, Angelique, Venomous Bites and Stings, Natural Remedies, 1993

Bulletin of Faculty of Pharmacy, Cairo University, "Umbelliferone: sources, Chemistry, and Bioactivities review" Internet, Science Direct, Volume 55, Issue 2, December 2017, pages 223-232

Buchman, Dian, Herbal Medicine, 1980

Caldicott, Helen, editor, Crises Without End, 2014, The New Press, New York, London

Cervoni, Barbie, RD, Kroner, Arno, DAOM, "Osha Root: What it is Good For." VerywellHealth.com, a medical board dedicated to providing up to date scientific information about medical diseases and issues.

Cordes, Betty, CRNA, Pocket Guide to Emergency First Aid, 2005, A pocket Guides publishing Book

Forgey, Wm, MD, Wilderness Medicine, 1987, ICS Books, INC

Herbal medicine, Expanded Commission E Monographs, 2000, Integrative Medicine Communications

IDEA, Health and Fitness Association, www.ideafit,com/fitness.com/library /fall prevention-program

Jarvis, D.C., MD, Folk Medicine, 1958

Kloss, Jethro, Back to Eden, 1971, Lancer Books

Moore, Michael S., Medicinal Plants of the Mountain West, 1979

Notes from classes and personal communication

PDR for Herbal Medicine, 4th edition, Thomas Healthcare Inc.,

Rodale's illustrated Encyclopedia of Herbs, 1987

Survival Wisdom& Know-How, Compiled by Amy Rost, Stackpole Books

Tso, Sam, Dineh herbalist, Personal communication

Werner David, Where There Is No Doctor, 1977, Hesperian Foundation

Wilderness Medicine Conference, Santa Fe, New Mexico, 2011

CALLING FOR HELP

When calling for help remain calm. Being hysterical delays help. Stay on the phone until the emergency dispatcher releases you from the call.

Information To Give 911 Operator Or Poison Control Center

NATIONAL POISON CONTROL CENTER: 1 800 222-1222

1. Exact location, address, and phone number. If there is no address or you don't know the address, look for landmarks, businesses, cross streets, prominent natural features.
2. Your name and victim's name if known.
3. The nature of the emergency and injury. Are there any animals involved?
4. Number of those involved.
5. Age and gender of victim and weight if known—or best estimate.
6. The victim:
    - b. Breathing?
    - c. Pulse?
    - d. Bleeding?
    - e. Level of response: Alert, awake, responds to name or noise, responds to pain only, no response?
7. For the alert victim: Ask "What bothers you the most?"

8. Obtain medical history:
    a. Diabetes
    b. Heart disease
    c. Allergies (especially to any medications)
    d. Time of last food or drink, and what was it?
    e. Are they wearing any medical jewelry?
9. If you suspect poison don't wait for symptoms to develop.
    a. Contact National Poison Control Center (PCC) immediately If you suspect poison. Don't wait for symptoms to develop. 1 800 222-1222.
    b. Don't guess what you should do.
    c. Time is of the essence and can make a difference between life or death.
    d. Try to determine what was ingested, how much and the time ingested.

Listed below are reasons for these reactions. Individual responses differ.

1. Misidentification of plant
2. Incorrect use of plant

FAMILY MEDICAL INFORMATION

NAME: ____

AGE: ____

BLOOD TYPE: ____

ALLERGIES & REACTIONS: ____________________________

____

OTHER MEDICAL INFORMATION; previous illnesses and operations, injuries, insect or animal bites requiring medical attention, family history, any recent exposures to infections_______________________________________

____

____

____

____

____

____

____

MEDICATIONS, VITAMINS, SUPPLEMENTS, HERBAL PRODUCTS TAKEN ON A DAILY BASIS, include dosages, this is especially important if taking insulin or diabetic medications____________________________________

____

____

____

DATE LAST TETANUS SHOT or booster

____

YOUR SPACE: THIS IS "YOUR" SPACE TO RECORD: DATE INCIDENT OCURED, TO WHOM DID IT OCUR, REMEDIES USED, OUTCOME, WHAT WORKED / WHAT DIDN'T WORK, WHAT WORKED FOR YOU.

ABOUT JESSIE EMERSON

Jessie Emerson has been a practicing registered nurse since 1965. In the 1970's she began to study holistic medicine. She graduated in 1989 from Michael Moore's Southwest School of Botanical Medicine and has studied with Native American herbalists, including Rolling Thunder and Navajo herbalist Sam Tso and Northern New Mexico Hispanic herbalists. She is the founder and owner of Oso Herbals. Oso Herbals and Jessie are dedicated to the respectful and correct use of the plant kingdom. OSO is the Spanish word for bear. "The bear came into my dreams and the bear and bear claw became the logo of my company and symbol of my medicine. The focus of Oso Herbals and Jessie is health, culture, the natural environment, and sustainability.

She has taken her first book Medicine From The Kitchen further to include plants that can easily be found in stores, the garden or in the backyard. Her goal for writing Nature to the Rescue is to empower people with knowledge that can prevent incidents, accidents, and injury and can help people remain calm during crises. She says, "It is my belief that we must know what to do when there is no doctor or what to do until medical help is available".

Jessie lives in a small town on the edge of the desert in New Mexico. She offers consultations, native medicinal plant tours, classes in medicine from the wild, and workshops in first aid using herbs, spices, and foods.

Contact Jessie at osoherbalsjessie@gmail.com

www.ingramcontent.com/pod-product-compliance
Lightning Source LLC
LaVergne TN
LVHW052323200926
848481LV00002B/649
* 9 7 9 8 8 6 8 9 0 7 4 6 3 *